ESSENTIAL ANATOMIES: ORAL AND HEAD/NECK

ESSENTIAL ANATOMIES:
Oral and Head/Neck

MARJORIE J. SHORT, R.D.H., B.S., M.S.
Middlesex Community College

with contributions by Deborah Levin-Goldstein, R.D.H., B.S., M.S.
Northampton County Area Community College

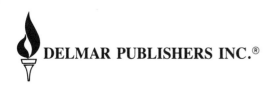
DELMAR PUBLISHERS INC.®

NOTICE TO THE READER

Publisher does not warrant or guarantee any of the products described herein or perform any independent analysis in connection with any of the product information contained herein. Publisher does not assume, and expressly disclaims, any obligation to obtain and include information other than that provided to it by the manufacturer.

The reader is expressly warned to consider and adopt all safety precautions that might be indicated by the activities described herein and to avoid all potential hazards. By following the instructions contained herein, the reader willingly assumes all risks in connection with such instructions.

The publisher makes no representations or warranties of any kind, including but not limited to, the warranties of fitness for particular purpose or merchantability, nor are any such representations implied with respect to the material set forth herein, and the publisher takes no responsibility with respect to such material. The publisher shall not be liable for any special, consequential or exemplary damages resulting, in whole or in part, from the readers' use of, or reliance upon, this material.

Delmar Staff
Administrative Editor: Leslie Boyer
Associate Editor: Karen Lavroff
Managing Editor: Barbara Christie
Production Editor: Ruth East
Design Coordinator: Susan Mathews

For information, address Delmar Publishers Inc.®
2 Computer Drive West, Box 15-015
Albany, New York 12212-9985

Printed in the United States of America
Published simultaneously in Canada
by Nelson Canada,
a division of International Thomson Limited

10   9   8   7   6   5   4   3   2   1

Library of Congress Cataloging in Publication Data

Short, Marjorie J., 1935-
  Essential anatomies.

  Bibliography: p.
  Includes index.
    1. Mouth—Anatomy. 2. Teeth—Anatomy. 3. Head—
Anatomy. 4. Neck—Anatomy. 5. Dental auxiliary person-
nel. I. Goldstein, Deborah Levin. II. Title.
[DNLM: 1. Head—anatomy & histology. 2. Neck—anatomy &
histology. 3. Tooth—anatomy & histology. WU 101 S559e]
QM306.S56   1987   611'.91   86-29038
ISBN 0-8273-2742-0 (pbk.)
ISBN 0-8273-2743-9 (instructor's guide)

Contents

SECTION TWO / PERMANENT ANTERIOR TEETH
Introductory Information

SECTION THREE / PERMANENT POSTERIOR TEETH
Introductory Information

SECTION FOUR / RELATED TOPICS

13
DECIDUOUS DENTITION   **140**

14
TOOTH DEVELOPMENT   **147**

15
OCCLUSION   **153**

16
FORM AND FUNCTION   **166**

SECTION FIVE / HEAD AND NECK ANATOMY

17
OSTEOLOGY OF THE SKULL   174

18
MUSCLES OF THE HEAD AND NECK   193

19
NERVES OF THE HEAD AND NECK   219

20
ARTERIES OF THE HEAD AND NECK   236

Preface

WHY THIS BOOK?

In the course of teaching dental auxiliaries, it became clear to the author that there was a need for a dental anatomy text that covered in depth the essential topics for an entry-level position in the dentist's office. As the role of the dental auxiliary broadens and becomes more important in providing dental services, our students need an understanding of basic theory and a way of relating that information to laboratory and clinical applications. In the past, instructors had to use books written for dental students, choosing a chapter from one, several paragraphs from another, and supplying the clinical applications themselves. ESSENTIAL ANATOMIES: ORAL AND HEAD/NECK meets the need for a single text. Written for the auxiliary, it presents the pertinent information in a concise, reasonably priced, and accessible format.

SPECIAL FEATURES

To that end, the book has several special features that enhance its usefulness to both the instructor and student.

- Outstanding Art Program. The book is extensively illustrated with exceptionally clear photographs and to-scale line drawings of teeth. Both normal and anomalous tooth development is depicted.

- Write-In Worksheets. Each chapter ends with a series of workbook-style worksheets that include review questions and exercises in identifying and labeling anatomical features and various aspects of the tooth.
- Tooth Identification Charts. Each tooth, in addition to being discussed in the context of the book, has its most important identifying features set off in a concise, brief chart. These charts are excellent for students to study from or refer to in clinical work.
- In-Text Student Aids. Objectives, Summaries, and Review Questions alert students to the most important concepts in each chapter, and help them recall and test their knowledge.

ACKNOWLEDGMENTS

To those who assisted me with this text, I extend my thanks and appreciation:

The American Dental Association, Chicago, Illinois, for contributing various illustrations,

Deborah Levin-Goldstein for her cooperation in the expansion of the text.

Allan M. Short, D.M.D., P.C., Assistant Clinical Instructor, Department of Orthodontics, Tufts University School of Dental Medicine, for his generous accommodation in editing the chapter on occlusion,

Leslie Boyer, Editor, and Ron Blackman, Art Director, for continual support and encouragement,

Kathy Bagay, Median School of Allied Health Careers; Janet Cassidy, Robert Morgan Vocational Institute; Janet Chernega, Fayetteville Technical Institute; Judith Cleary, New York University Dental Center; Lynn Cone, McCann Technical School; Diane Davis, Bakersfield College; Mark Knutsen, Miami-Dade Community College; Marion McCullough, El Centro College; and Karen Waide, Portland Community College for insightful and instructive reviews of the manuscript in various stages.

INTRODUCTION TO THE ORAL CAVITY

1

Nomenclature

THE DENTITION
THE NAMES AND FUNCTIONS OF THE TEETH
THE ARRANGEMENT OF THE TEETH
THE ERUPTION SEQUENCE

Objectives

- Identify, by name, the two dental arches, the permanent teeth, the deciduous teeth, and anterior and posterior teeth.
- Describe the order in which the teeth are positioned in the dental arch, the function of each type of tooth, and the eruption sequence of deciduous and permanent teeth.
- Define the terms noted in italics.
- Complete the worksheets at the end of the chapter.

THE DENTITION

Teeth are arranged in the jaws to form two dental arches. Each arch is named to correspond with the bone from which it is composed. The maxilla forms the maxillary or upper arch; the mandible forms the mandibular or lower arch. Together, the two arches make up one *dentition*, or set of teeth, Figure 1-1. During a lifespan, each person will have two dentitions, the deciduous and the permanent.

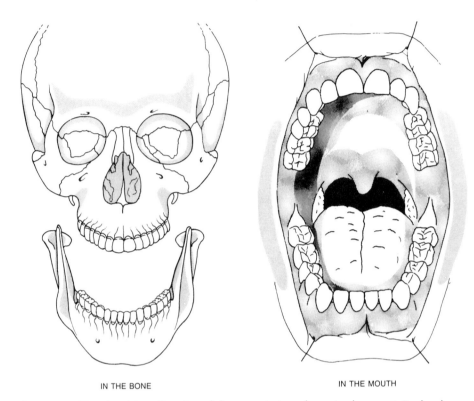

IN THE BONE   IN THE MOUTH

Figure 1-1 The dentition (Reprinted, by permission, from Anderson & Burkard, *The Dental Assistant*, Figs. 4–1 and 9–1. © 1982 by Delmar Publishers, Inc.)

The Deciduous Dentition

The first or primary set of teeth, the deciduous dentition, begins to emerge into the mouth between 6–8 months of age. Teeth continue to erupt periodically, following a developmental schedule, until 20 teeth, 10 maxillary and 10 mandibular, have erupted by the age of 2½–3 years. These 20 deciduous teeth are small, but they fulfill the needs of a child. As the child grows, the deciduous teeth eventually *exfoliate*, or shed, and are replaced by permanent teeth. When all the permanent teeth have erupted, by the ages of 17 through 21, the permanent dentition is complete.

The Permanent Dentition

There are 32 permanent teeth, 16 maxillary and 16 mandibular. Until the child is 5 years old, only deciduous teeth are present in the mouth. Between 5 and 6 years of age, the first permanent tooth, the mandibular first molar, erupts posterior to the last deciduous molar. No deciduous tooth has exfoliated to provide space for this permanent tooth; however, the mandible has increased in length so that there is now space for an additional tooth. Permanent molars do not replace or succeed deciduous teeth.

Shortly after the permanent first molars erupt, deciduous incisors, the front teeth, begin to exfoliate. This occurs as a result of a physiological process that causes their roots to resorb as the permanent teeth form in the bone directly beneath them. Eventually, every deciduous tooth will exfoliate and be succeeded by a permanent tooth.

Between the ages of 5 and 12, some deciduous and permanent teeth are both present in the mouth at the same time; this is referred to as a *mixed dentition*. Permanent teeth that replace or succeed deciduous teeth are called *succedaneous* teeth and include incisors, canines, and premolars. Permanent molars are not succedaneous teeth because they do not replace deciduous teeth.

Because human beings have two successive sets of teeth during their lives (a deciduous and a permanent dentition), they are considered *diphyodonts*. Having several sets of teeth throughout life, such as certain reptiles do, would make the species *polyphyodonts*.

THE NAMES AND FUNCTIONS OF THE TEETH

Each dentition includes several types of teeth shaped to perform specific functions. People are *heterodonts* because they have different types of teeth called incisors, canines, premolars, and molars. The types of teeth in the maxillary arch are the same as those in the mandibular arch. When an imaginary midline is drawn to divide the arches into a right and left quadrant, the teeth in the right quadrant are the same as those in the left quadrant.

The Permanent Teeth

As mentioned before, the permanent dentition has 32 teeth, 16 maxillary and 16 mandibular, Figure 1-2. They are listed on page 6.

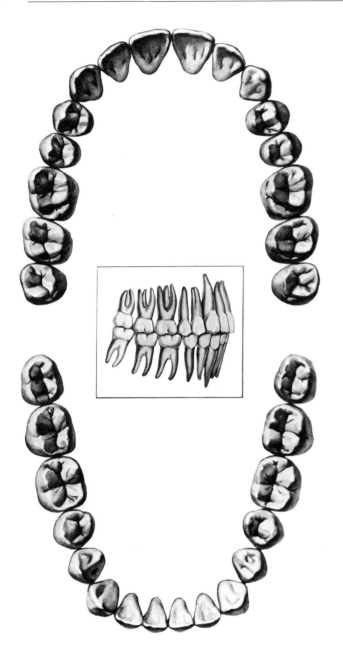

Figure 1-2 The permanent dentition
(Copyright by the American Dental Association.
Reprinted by permission.)

Types of Teeth	**Number per arch**
Incisors are the four front teeth and have sharp biting edges for incising, or cutting, food. The two in the middle of the arch are central incisors; those on either side are lateral incisors.	4
Canines are the corner teeth and have one pointed cusp used to hold and tear food.	2
Premolars are posterior teeth having two major cusps adapted to crush and tear food. Premolars are named by their sequence in the arch from front to back as "first premolar" and "second premolar."	4
Molars are broad back teeth having several cusps adapted to chew, crush, and grind food. They, too, are named by their sequence from the front to the back of the arch as "first molar," "second molar," and "third molar."	6
By working together, each tooth performing its individual function in the process of *mastication*, or chewing, the food is prepared for swallowing and digestion.	16 Total per arch

The Deciduous Teeth

The deciduous dentition (as mentioned earlier) has 20 teeth, 10 maxillary and 10 mandibular, Figure 1-3. They are smaller but similar in shape and function to the permanent teeth. They are as follows:

Types of Teeth	**Number in Arch**
Incisors — two central and two lateral	4
Canines — one in each corner of the arch	2
Molars — two first molars, two second molars	4
Each deciduous tooth is eventually replaced by a permanent tooth. Note, however, that there are no deciduous premolars. Deciduous molars are succeeded by permanent premolars.	10 Total per arch

Each deciduous tooth is eventually replaced by a permanent tooth. Note, however, that there are no deciduous premolars. Deciduous molars are succeeded by permanent premolars. Permanent molars erupt posterior to the deciduous molars without replacing any deciduous teeth. As mentioned before, permanent molars are not succedaneous teeth.

THE ARRANGEMENT OF THE TEETH

Figure 1-2 shows the arrangement of the teeth in the dental arches. The *anterior* teeth are those in the front of the mouth and include incisors and canines. *Posterior* teeth, those in the back of the mouth, include premolars and molars.

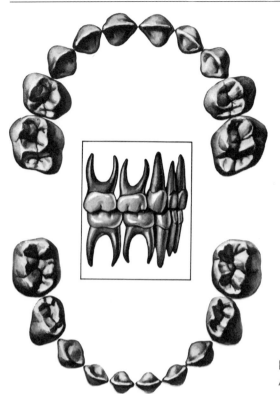

Figure 1-3 The deciduous dentition (Copyright by the American Dental Association. Reprinted by permission.)

Tooth Description

To identify a tooth correctly it is designated not only by its name and arch but by the quadrant in which it is located. Each quadrant is specified according to the patient's right or left side. To completely identify a tooth, information is given in the following sequence:

	DENTITION	ARCH	QUADRANT	TOOTH
example	Permanent	Mandibular	Right	Incisor

THE ERUPTION SEQUENCE

Although teeth begin to form in utero, they do not begin to erupt until 6–8 months of age. Eruption dates vary from person to person by a few months, just as the individual growth rate varies. Following is the eruption sequence for *deciduous teeth*. Note that mandibular teeth generally precede maxillary teeth in eruption.

TOOTH	MONTHS (±)
Mandibular central incisors	6
Mandibular lateral incisors	7
Maxillary central incisors	7½
Maxillary lateral incisors	8
Mandibular first molars	12-16
Maxillary first molars	14
Mandibular canines	16
Maxillary canines	18
Mandibular second molars	20
Maxillary second molars	24

By the age of 2½–3 years, all deciduous teeth have erupted; at about 6 years, the permanent teeth start to erupt. Refer to Figure 1-4 for the growth pattern of the teeth. A chronology of this growth pattern is given in Appendix A.

    The first molars are the first permanent teeth to emerge into the mouth. They erupt posterior to the deciduous second molar without replacing any deciduous teeth. The eruption sequence of the *permanent dentition* is as follows:

TOOTH	YEARS (±)
Mandibular first molars	6-7
Maxillary first molars	6-7
Mandibular central incisors	6-7
Mandibular lateral incisors	7-8
Maxillary central incisors	7-8
Maxillary lateral incisors	8-9
Mandibular canines	9-10
Maxillary first premolars	10-11
Mandibular first premolars	10-12
Maxillary second premolars	11-12
Mandibular second premolars	11-12
Maxillary canines	11-12
Mandibular second molars	11-13
Maxillary second molars	12-13
Third molars	17-21

DEVELOPMENT OF THE HUMAN DENTITION

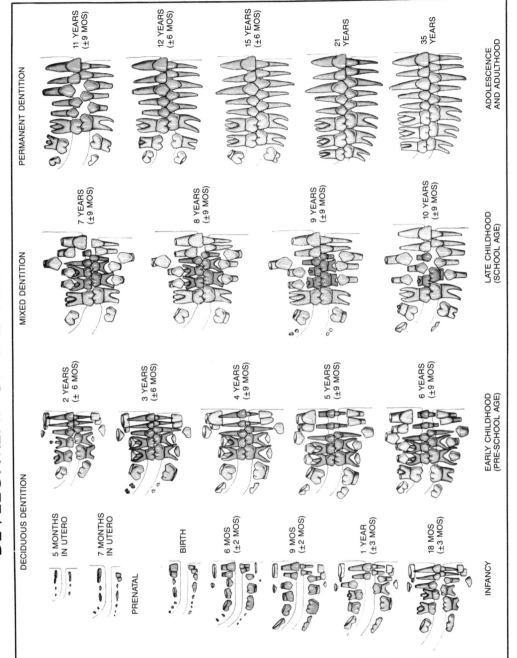

Figure 1-4 Development of human dentitions (Copyright by the American Dental Association. Reprinted by permission.)

The initial eruption period, called *active eruption*, continues until the crown is almost completely exposed and the tooth is in its proper alignment. In later life, the "gums," or gingival line, may recede, exposing more of the tooth. This process is referred to as *passive eruption*.

Continual use of the teeth throughout life can cause a slight wearing away of the biting and/or chewing surfaces, and thus a decrease in the height of the tooth. This wearing away is called *attrition*. Grinding of the teeth (bruxism) also causes attrition. *Abrasion* of the tooth surfaces can be caused by mechanical wear such as continual biting on an object or brushing too vigorously.

SUMMARY

During a person's lifespan there will be two sets of teeth. The first set, the primary or deciduous dentition, consists of 20 teeth. It eventually exfoliates and is replaced by the permanent dentition, which has 32 teeth.

Each dentition has several types of teeth shaped to perform a specific function; they work in conjunction with each other to prepare the food for digestion.

Deciduous teeth begin to emerge during the sixth month of infancy, but are not completely erupted as a full dentition until the third year of life. Permanent teeth begin to emerge between five and six years of age, and all but the third molars will have erupted by the twelfth year. Permanent teeth are expected to last a lifetime.

WORKSHEET

A. Define the following words.

Active eruption _____

Anterior _____

Attrition _____

Deciduous _____

Dentition _____

Diphyodont _____

Exfoliate _____

Heterodont _____

Mastication _____

Passive Eruption _____

Polyphyodont _____

Posterior _____

Succedaneous _____

B. Complete the following information.

   1. The following illustration represents the biting surfaces of the deciduous maxillary dentition. Label the teeth of the right quadrant.

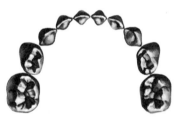

   2. The following illustration represents the biting surfaces of the permanent maxillary dentition. Label the teeth of the left quadrant.

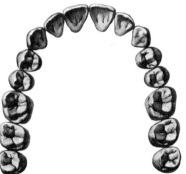

3. Using the illustrations on page 11, circle the posterior teeth of the deciduous dentition—left quadrant
permanent dentition—right quadrant

4. Using the following illustrations, number the teeth in their correct eruption sequence.

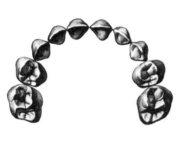
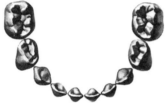
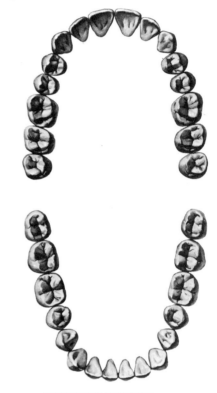

DECIDUOUS DENTITION   PERMANENT DENTITION

2
Structures of the Oral Cavity

RELATED TERMINOLOGY
THE ORAL CAVITY
EXTERNAL STRUCTURES OF THE ORAL CAVITY
STRUCTURES OF THE ORAL VESTIBULE
STRUCTURES OF THE ORAL CAVITY PROPER

Objectives

- Identify two areas of the oral cavity, the boundaries of the oral vestibule, and the boundaries of the oral cavity proper.
- Describe each structure of the oral cavity as to location, color, size, and/or shape.
- Define the terms noted in italics.
- Complete the worksheets at the end of the chapter.

RELATED TERMINOLOGY

The names of many oral cavity structures, as well as associated and descriptive terms, are derived from Latin words. Since these words appear over and over again throughout the readings it is helpful to become familiar with them.

Alba . . . . white
Bucca . . . . cheek
Buccal . . . . relating to the cheek

Fornix . . . . arch
Frenum . . . . folds of tissue
Labia . . . . lip
Labial . . . . relating to the lip
Linea . . . . line
Lingual . . . . relating to the tongue
Mental . . . . relating to the chin
Nasal . . . . relating to the nose
Naso . . . . nose
Oral . . . . relating to the mouth
Plica . . . . fold (of tissue)
Raphe . . . . a seam (of tissue)
Sub . . . . under

THE ORAL CAVITY

The term "oral cavity" is used when referring to the inner portion of the mouth. The oral cavity extends from the anterior opening at the lips to the posterior border, the oro-pharynx, or throat. The palate, or roof of the mouth, is the superior border and the tongue, along with the musculature beneath it, defines the inferior or lower boundary.

A soft, moist tissue called the *mucous membrane* lines the oral cavity. In the mouth, the mucous membrane is referred to as the *oral mucosa*. Oral mucosa is pink and occurs in various degrees of thickness. Although not as strong or as thick as skin, it acts as a protective covering for the oral cavity. In some areas the oral mucosa is firmly attached, as on the gingiva and hard palate. In other areas, such as the cheek, it is much looser. There are three types of oral mucosa, each classified according to function and location:

1. Masticatory mucosa covers areas subject to stress such as gingival tissue and the hard palate.

2. Specialized mucosa covers the area that has a specific function of taste on the dorsum of the tongue.

3. Lining mucosa covers all other areas of the oral cavity such as the inner surfaces of the lips and cheeks, and the floor and roof of the mouth.

Divisions

The oral cavity is divided into two sections, the oral vestibule and the oral cavity proper. The *oral vestibule* is the area between the inner lips and cheeks (buccal mucosa) and the front (facial) surfaces of the teeth. The *oral cavity proper* extends from the inner (lingual) surfaces of the teeth to the oro-pharynx.

Functions

Chewing of food, or mastication, is the most obvious function of the oral cavity. As chewing occurs, food is moistened with saliva, preparing it for swallowing (deglutition) and digestion. The tongue provides taste for the food and assists the cheek and lip muscles with movement of food around the oral cavity. In addition to these functions, the oral cavity provides an air passage and assists the tongue with speech.

EXTERNAL STRUCTURES OF THE ORAL CAVITY

The structures of the lips, cheeks, and related areas of the face are closely associated with the oral cavity because they assist with its effective functioning, Figure 2-1. These outer structures are made up of muscles that aid in opening and closing the lips, and compressing food against as well as moving it away from the teeth. They include:

Labial commissure: the closure line of the lips

Philtrum: a shallow depression extending from the area below the middle of the nose to the center of the upper lip

Vermilion area: the pink zone of the lips

Naso-labial sulcus: a shallow depression extending from the corner of the nose to the corner of the lips

Labio-mental groove: a shallow linear depression between the center of the lower lip and the chin

Labio-marginal sulcus: a shallow depression extending downward from the corners of the mouth

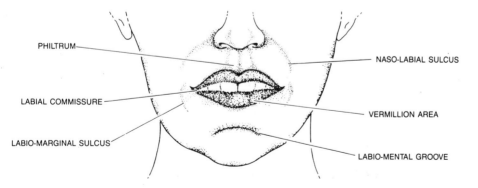

Figure 2-1 External structures associated with the oral cavity

STRUCTURES OF THE ORAL VESTIBULE

Although the oral vestibule is a small antechamber, it contains several structures that should be recognized, Figure 2-2.

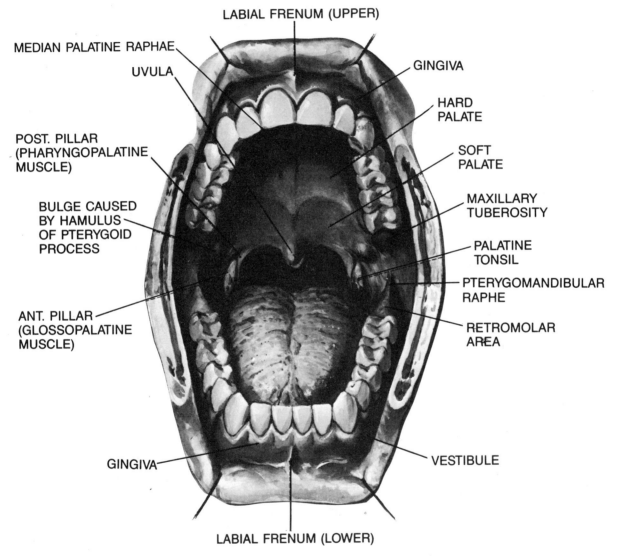

Figure 2-2 Structures of the oral cavity (Copyright by the American Dental Association. Reprinted by permission.)

Labial frenum: an elevated fold of soft mucous tissue extending from the alveolar mucosa of the two central incisors to the labial mucosa (A superior frenum exists in the maxillary area; an inferior frenum is located in the mandibular area.)

Buccal frenum: an elevated fold of soft tissue extending from the alveolar mucosa above the canine or premolar to the buccal mucosa

Boney eminence: a raised contour of bone, covered with soft tissue, that follows the roots of the tooth

Maxillary tuberosity: a small, rounded extension of bone, covered with soft tissue, posterior to the last maxillary tooth .

Retromolar area: a triangular area of bone, covered with soft tissue, posterior to the last mandibular tooth

Stensen's papilla: a small, raised flap of soft tissue on the buccal mucosa opposite the maxillary molar (It is often marked with a tiny red dot which is the opening to the parotid or Stensen's salivary gland.)

Linea alba: a raised, white horizontal extension of soft tissue along the buccal mucosa at the occlusal line (The literal translation of these words is "white line." The linea alba is not present in all mouths.)

Gingiva: pink, stippled mucosa surrounding the necks of the teeth and covering the bone in which the teeth are anchored

Fordyce granules: small, yellow spots on the buccal mucosa and inner lip. They are sebaceous glands and have no clinical significance.

STRUCTURES OF THE ORAL CAVITY PROPER

When the mouth is wide open, it is possible to observe all the structures of the oral cavity proper. The following structures are located on the roof of the mouth (see Figure 2-3):

Palate: the concave surface that is known as the roof of the mouth and is divided into the hard and soft palate

Hard palate: the boney anterior ⅔ of the palate that is covered with mucosa

Soft palate: the posterior third of the palate, made up of muscular fibers covered with mucosa (It is a deeper color pink than the hard palate because of its highly vascular composition.)

Palatine torus: a boney prominence of varied size located at the midline of the hard palate (It is a nonpathological excess of bone covered with mucosa and is only present in about 20 percent of the population.)

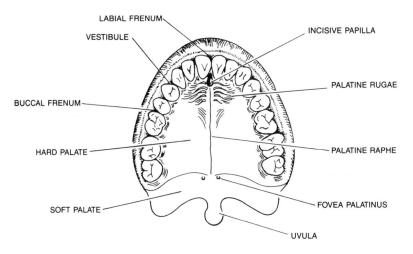

Figure 2-3 Structures on the roof of the mouth

Incisive papilla: a small, raised, rounded structure of soft tissue at the anterior midline of the hard palate (It is directly behind the two maxillary central incisors and covers and protects the incisive foramen, an opening in the bone directly beneath it through which nerves and blood vessels travel.)

Palatine raphe: a junction of soft tissue extending the entire midline of the hard palate

Palatine rugae: paired transverse, palatine folds of soft tissue on the anterior portion of the hard palate (The rugae extend horizontally to keep the food from adhering to the palate.)

Fovea palatinus: two small indentations, one on either side of the raphe, located at the junction of the hard and soft palate (These are remnants of minor salivary glands. Their only value is as the terminal demarcation in the fabrication of a maxillary denture.)

Uvula: a downward projection of the soft palate made up of connective tissue, muscles, and glands

The following structures are located at the posterior portion of the oral cavity and form the pillars of fauces, the arch or entryway that joins the oral cavity with the pharynx.

Oro-pharynx: the area of the oral cavity that joins it with the throat or pharynx (On either side are the arches of muscular tissue called the *pillars of fauces*.)

Glossopalatine muscle: the anterior pillar of fauces extending from the outer surface of the palate to the tongue

Pharyngopalatine muscle: the posterior pillar of fauces extending from the pharynx to the palate

Palatine tonsils: masses of lymphoid tissue located between the anterior and posterior pillars of fauces

The following structures are located on the floor of the oral cavity proper. In order for them to be observed, the tongue must be raised as shown in Figure 2-4.

Tongue: a muscular structure covered with oral mucosa and papillae that contains taste buds.

Lingual Frenum: an elevated fold of soft tissue located on the floor of the mouth at the midline. It extends from the tissue below the central incisors to the undersurface of the tongue.

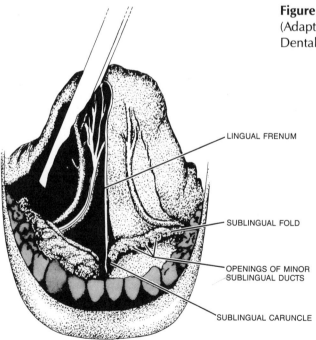

Figure 2-4 Structures on the floor of the mouth (Adapted from a figure copyrighted by the American Dental Association. Used by permission.)

LINGUAL FRENUM

SUBLINGUAL FOLD

OPENINGS OF MINOR
SUBLINGUAL DUCTS

SUBLINGUAL CARUNCLE

Sublingual Caruncles: round, elevated sections of soft tissue on either side of the lingual frenum, directly behind the central incisors on the floor of the mouth. Within the caruncles are duct openings to the sublingual (Wharton's) and sub-maxillary (Bartholin's) salivary glands.

Sublingual Plica: an elevated fold of soft tissue extending, medially, along the floor of the mouth toward the tongue. This fold contains the opening to salivary glands called the *Ducts of Rivinus.*

Mandibular Tori: an overgrowth of bone occurring bilaterally on the internal borders of the mandible. As with the maxillary torus, they are nonpathological and occur in only 8 percent of the population.

SUMMARY

The oral cavity, or mouth, is lined with a soft, moist covering called the *oral mucosa.* The lining has different degrees of consistency that enhance and protect oral structures such as the tongue and hard palate.

The external structures of the oral cavity include the lips, cheeks, and related areas of the face that assist the oral cavity to function effectively.

It is important to be familiar with the complete anatomy of the oral structures as well as with the terminology necessary for differentiating normal from abnormal.

WORKSHEET

A. Define the following terms.

Buccal _____

Deglutition _____

Frenum_____

Labial _____

Lingual _____

Mental _____

Nasal _____

Plica _____

Raphe _____

B. Complete the following.

1. The two major areas of the oral cavity are _____ and _____.

2. The boundaries of the oral cavity are:

   Laterally— _____

   Anteriorly— _____

   Posteriorly— _____

   Superiorly— _____

   Inferiorly— _____

3. The vestibule is the space between the inner lip and cheeks and _____.

4. The fauces form the opening from the oral cavity into the _____.

5. The portion of the oral mucosa that surrounds the neck of the tooth is the _____.

C. Label the following diagrams.

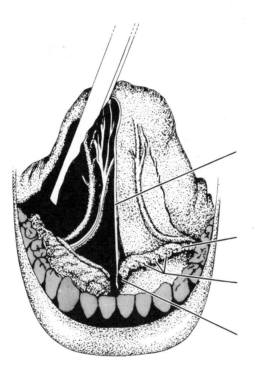

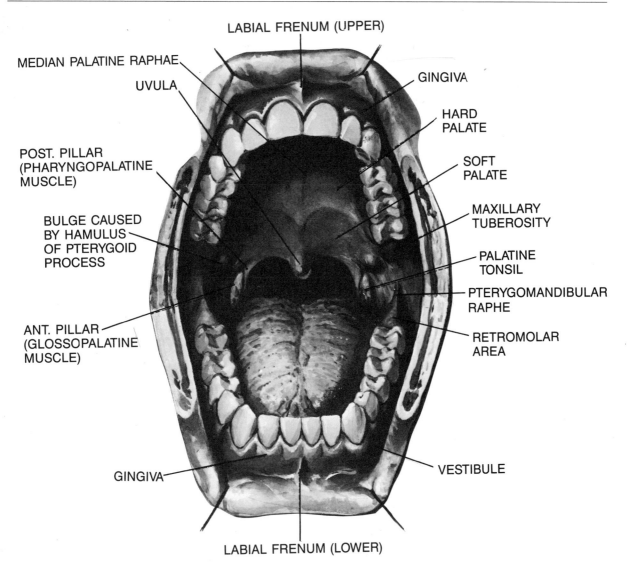

LABIAL FRENUM (UPPER)

MEDIAN PALATINE RAPHAE

UVULA

GINGIVA

HARD PALATE

POST. PILLAR (PHARYNGOPALATINE MUSCLE)

SOFT PALATE

BULGE CAUSED BY HAMULUS OF PTERYGOID PROCESS

MAXILLARY TUBEROSITY

PALATINE TONSIL

PTERYGOMANDIBULAR RAPHE

ANT. PILLAR (GLOSSOPALATINE MUSCLE)

RETROMOLAR AREA

GINGIVA

VESTIBULE

LABIAL FRENUM (LOWER)

D. Describe the following structures as to location, color, size, and/or shape.

Labial Commissure _____

Naso-labial Sulcus _____

Philtrum _____

Maxillary Tuberosity _____

Retromolar Area _____

Frenum _____

Incisive Papilla _____

Palatine Rugae _____

Palatine Raphe _____

Fovea Palatinus _____

Pillars of Fauces _____

Uvula _____

Stenson's Papilla _____

Sublingual Plica _____

Sublingual Caruncle _____

Palatine Tonsils _____

Vermilion Area _____

3

The Tooth and Its Surrounding Structures

DIVISIONS OF THE TOOTH
SURFACES OF THE TOOTH
TISSUES OF THE TOOTH
THE PERIODONTIUM

Objectives
- Identify the divisions of the tooth, the surfaces of the tooth, tissues of the tooth, and tissues of the periodontium.
- Describe each tooth tissue and those of the surrounding structures as to location, composition, and function.
- Define the terms noted in italics.
- Complete the worksheets at the end of the chapter.

DIVISIONS OF THE TOOTH

To examine the tooth it is divided into three sections (Figure 3-1):
    1. the crown
    2. the neck or cervix
    3. the root

The *crown* is that portion of the tooth normally visible in the mouth and covered with enamel. The teeth have differently shaped crowns, each adapted to perform a specific function in reducing food for digestion.

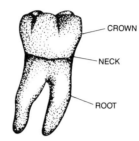

Figure 3-1 Divisions of the tooth

The *root*, located in the bone and not normally visible, is covered with cementum. Roots stabilize, or support, the teeth when the pressure from mastication is exerted upon them. The crown joins the root at the neck, *cervix*, or cemento-enamel junction (CEJ), a junction between the *anatomical crown* and the *anatomical root*. The anatomical crown is covered with enamel; the anatomical root is covered with cementum. After eruption is complete, only the anatomical crown is seen in the mouth. In later life, as part of the aging process, the gingiva and bone may recede, exposing a portion of the root. All of the tooth that is visible in the mouth, the crown *and* the exposed root together, is referred to as the *clinical crown*.

SURFACES OF THE TOOTH

Every tooth has five surfaces, each surface named according to its position in the arch, Figure 3-2.

Mesial: the surface closest to the midline

Distal: the surface farthest, or most distant, from the midline

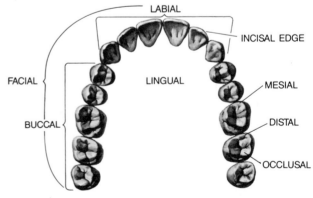

Figure 3-2 Surfaces of the teeth
(Base art copyright by the American Dental Association. Reprinted by permission.)

Facial: the surfaces closest to the face or outer surfaces of the teeth, including

   Labial: facial surfaces of anterior teeth or surfaces closest to the lip

   Buccal: facial surfaces of posterior teeth or surfaces closest to the cheek

Lingual: surfaces closest to the tongue; all the inner surfaces

Occlusal: chewing surfaces of the posterior teeth

Incisal edge: biting surface of the anterior teeth

Other terms that relate to the surfaces of the teeth are:

Proximal: the surface of the tooth that is next to, or beside, the adjacent tooth (Mesial and distal surfaces are both proximal surfaces.)

Interproximal area: a triangular space between adjacent teeth that is normally filled with the portion of the gingiva called interdental papilla

Contact area: an area on both the mesial and distal surfaces that touches, or contacts, the adjacent tooth

Apex: the tip of the root

Line angle: the area of the tooth where two surfaces meet (For example, the line that joins the buccal and mesial surfaces, Figure 3-3.)

Point angle: the area of the tooth where three surfaces meet (For example, the joining point of the occlusal, lingual, and mesial surfaces shown in Figure 3-3.)

To describe the precise location of an anatomical tooth structure, it is useful to divide the crown and root into thirds as shown in Figure 3–4. Imaginary horizontal lines divide the crown into incisal or occlusal, middle, and cervical thirds and

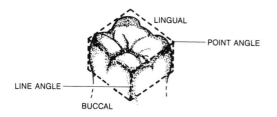

Figure 3-3 Point and line angles

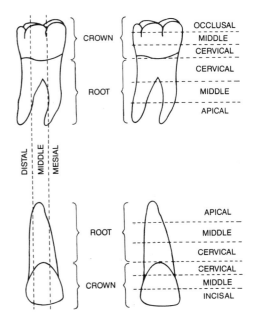

Figure 3-4 Vertical thirds/horizontal thirds

the root into cervical, middle, and apical thirds. Vertical thirds can be used to divide the tooth into mesial, middle, and distal thirds also shown in Figure 3-4. When explaining details of the tooth a groove can be described as extending to the junction of the occlusal and middle third. This same groove can be located in the distal third of the tooth.

TISSUES OF THE TOOTH

The tissues of the teeth are shown in Figure 3-5 and described below.

Enamel
The crown of the tooth is covered with enamel, the hardest tissue in the body. Enamel is made up of 96 percent inorganic (mineral) and 4 percent organic matter and water. It varies in thickness from 2 to 2.5 mm at the biting surface of the tooth to a very thin layer near the cervix. Microscopically, the enamel is made up of millions of tiny enamel rods extending from the dentin outwardly, to form the framework of the tooth. Once enamel is complete, it cannot be increased or

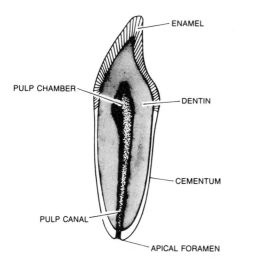

Figure 3-5 Tissues of the tooth

decreased by a physiological forming process. However, it is subject to attrition and dental decay, external processes that occur after the tooth has erupted. Because of its density, enamel is the protective layer of the tooth.

Cementum

Cementum covers the root of the tooth and has the same density as bone. It is 50 percent inorganic and 50 percent organic matter and water. Cementum forms a very thin layer over the root, 0.05 mm or no thicker than a coat of paint on a wall, resulting in its being easily removed during scaling or root planing, or by abrasion when the root is exposed. However, additional cementum can be produced after the eruption of the tooth on areas not exposed in the oral cavity.

Theoretically, the cementum joins the enamel at the cemento-enamel junction. Histologically, however, one of three variations can occur at the cervix:

1. The cementum slightly overlaps the enamel, the most commonly occurring condition.
2. The cementum joins smoothly with enamel.
3. A tiny gap exists between the cementum and the enamel.

Cementum attaches the tooth to the bone by tiny fibers called Sharpey's fibers. These extend from the surrounding periodontal ligament into the cementum.

Dentin

Dentin makes up the major portion of both the crown and the root of the tooth. It is located directly beneath the enamel of the crown and the cementum of the root. Dentin, harder than bone, is 70 percent inorganic and 30 percent organic matter and water. It is made up of an organic matrix which contains dentinal tubules. The tubules are filled with dentinal fibrils that extend from the pulp to the enamel and carry sensation (temperature, pain) to the pulp.

Pulp

The pulp is located at the innermost portion of the tooth and is the only soft tissue of the tooth. It is made up of blood vessels, cellular substances, and nerves.

That portion of the pulp located in the crown is the *pulp chamber*. It conforms to the shape of the crown, forming small peaks, or *pulp horns*, on the posterior teeth where the crown rises to form cusps, Figure 3-6. The pulp canal is the portion of the pulp located in the root of the tooth. Together, the pulp chamber and the pulp canal occupy the *pulp cavity*, a space within the center of the tooth. Vessels of the pulp enter and exit the tooth through a small apical *foramen*, or hole, in the apex of the root where they merge with other similar vessels of the jaw.

The function of the pulp is to assist in the production of dentin, provide sensitivity to the tooth, and act as a defense mechanism by reacting to injury. It also provides nourishment to the tooth.

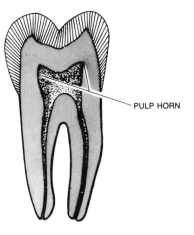

Figure 3-6 The pulp horn

THE PERIODONTIUM

The periodontium includes those structures that surround and support the teeth (Figure 3-7):

- cementum
- periodontal ligament
- alveolar process
- gingiva

Cementum

Cementum, previously described as a tissue of the tooth, is also considered a supporting structure because it contains fibers from the periodontal ligament that hold the tooth in its socket.

Periodontal Ligament

The periodontal ligament surrounds the root of the tooth. It is made up of fibers, or ligaments, that support and suspend the tooth in the *alveolus*, or socket. Like

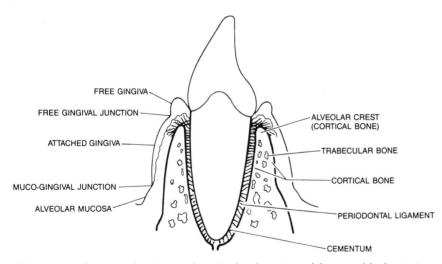

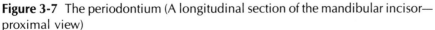

Figure 3-7 The periodontium (A longitudinal section of the mandibular incisor—proximal view)

a tiny trampoline, the fibers, arranged in bundles, act as a shock absorber to keep the tooth from pushing against the bone during the extreme pressure resulting from mastication. Other fibers extend from the periodontal ligament into the cementum on one side and into the alveolar process on the other side to attach the tooth to the bone. These are Sharpey's fibers.

Besides the fibers, the periodontal ligament contains nerves, blood, and lymph vessels. Its function is to produce cementum; stimulate bone resorption; provide sensation upon pressure to the tooth; and provide nutrients through the blood vessels.

Alveolar Process

The alveolar process is that portion of the maxilla and mandible that surrounds the roots of the teeth. It is separated from the roots by the periodontal ligament and is made up of bone tissue composed of two layers:

1. cancellous or trabecular bone
2. compact or cortical bone

The inner layer, lightweight and porous, is the trabecular bone. It is surrounded by a denser layer of compact bone structured to endure stress. Compact bone is located adjacent to the periodontal ligament and at the alveolar crest. The layer that surrounds the periodontal ligament forms the socket or *alveolus* of each tooth and is called the lamina dura, meaning hard layer.

Cancellous bone, the innermost layer, is less dense because of the tiny spaces called trabeculae. Without these trabeculae to provide porousness, the bone would be too heavy to move.

The alveolar process supports the tooth and stabilizes the root.

Gingiva

Gingiva, the only portion of the periodontium visible in the oral cavity, is made up of epithelial tissue covered with mucosa, Figure 3-8. It attaches to the underlying bone, surrounds the cervix of the tooth, and fills the interproximal space. It is divided into two sections, free or marginal gingiva and attached gingiva.

Free Gingiva. The gingiva that surrounds the cervix (neck) of the tooth is like a collar and fills the interproximal spaces where it forms the interdental papilla.

Free or marginal gingiva is unattached on the inner surface creating a space or tiny gingival sulcus between it and the tooth, as shown in Figure 3-9. The depth of the gingival sulcus is about 1.2 to 1.8 mm before it reaches the epithelial attachment, a layer of cells that merge it with the tooth and the attached gingiva.

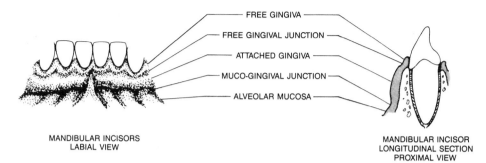

FREE GINGIVA

FREE GINGIVAL JUNCTION

ATTACHED GINGIVA

MUCO-GINGIVAL JUNCTION

ALVEOLAR MUCOSA

MANDIBULAR INCISORS
LABIAL VIEW

MANDIBULAR INCISOR
LONGITUDINAL SECTION
PROXIMAL VIEW

Figure 3-8 Divisions of the gingiva

The gingival sulcus forms a tiny triangle between the free gingiva and the surface of the tooth as its sides, the epithelial attachment as the apex.

Attached gingiva. The portion of the gingiva that can be observed on the external surface. It merges with the free gingiva at the *free gingival junction*, a slight demarcation about 1.2 to 1.8 mm from the gingival crest. The attached gingiva extends apically from the free gingival junction, adhering tightly to the bone beneath it. As compared to other sections of the gingiva, it is pale pink because it is taut to the bone and contains less blood vessels.

Attached gingiva extends apically 3.5 to 9.0 mm where it merges with the *alveolar mucosa* at the *muco-gingival junction*, a scalloped line that follows the contour of the bone.

Figure 3-9 The gingival sulcus

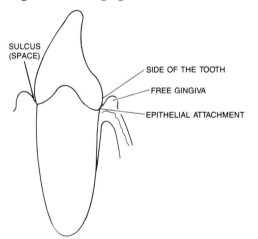

SULCUS
(SPACE)

SIDE OF THE TOOTH

FREE GINGIVA

EPITHELIAL ATTACHMENT

Gingival description. Gingiva is pink and stippled (like the skin of an orange) on the attached portion. The color varies with the skin pigmentation so that the darker the skin, the deeper the pink of the gingiva. Occasionally dark patches of pigmentation, *melanin,* appear on the gingiva of a darker skinned person; these spots of color are normal.

Gingiva is firm and resilient; it follows the contour of the bone and fills the interproximal spaces forming a sharp, knifelike triangular point at the contact area. Attached gingiva adheres tightly to the bone and is pale, compared to the smooth shiny alveolar mucosa which contains many blood vessels and thus appears more red in color.

SUMMARY

The integrity of the tooth depends on the good health and stability of all the periodontal tissues. Together, they provide and maintain the longevity of the dentition and protect it from injury.

WORKSHEET

A. Using the following drawing, answer the questions.

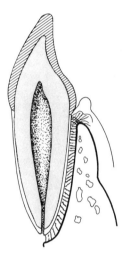

1. Name the boundaries of the gingival sulcus and label these boundaries on the illustration with numerals a, b, c.

   a. _____ b. _____ c._____

2. Name the two hard tissues into which the periodontal ligament fibers insert. Label d, e.

   d. _____ e. _____

3. Name the hardest and the least hard of the calcified tissues of the tooth. Label f, g.

   f._____ g. _____

4. Name the two divisions of the gingiva and the line of demarcation between them. Label h, i, j.
   h. _____ i._____ j. _____

5. Indicate the location of the pulp chamber by labeling it k.

6. Differentiate between the anatomical crown (label l) and the clinical crown (label m). Draw the cervical line.

B. Using the following drawing, label the structures listed below.

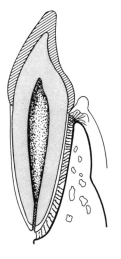

a. Enamel
b. Dentin
c. Pulp canal
d. Cementum
e. Apical foramen

f. Periodontal ligament
g. Cortical bone
h. Trabecular bone
i. Alveolar crest
j. Muco-gingival junction

4

Numbering Systems

THE UNIVERSAL NUMBERING SYSTEM
PALMER'S NOTATION
FEDERATION DENTAIRE INTERNATIONALE (FDI)

Objectives

- Identify three different numbering systems.
- Describe each numbering system as to its designation of dentition, arch, quadrant, and tooth.
- Complete the worksheets at the end of the chapter.

THE UNIVERSAL NUMBERING SYSTEM

Permanent Teeth

In the United States, the Universal Numbering System is the most widely accepted method used to record teeth. It is uncomplicated and efficient. Each tooth is numbered from 1 to 32 in consecutive order beginning with the patient's maxillary right third molar as tooth #1 and continuing to the maxillary left third molar, tooth #16, Figure 4-1. The numbers continue on the mandibular left side, #17 — the mandibular left third molar, and follow consecutively to the mandibular right third molar, tooth #32.

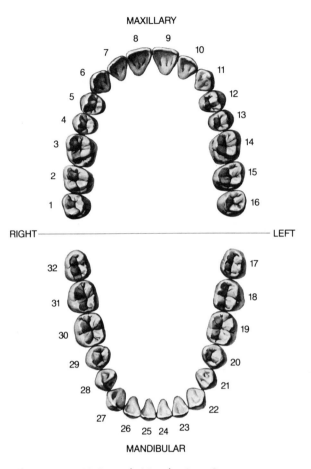

Figure 4-1 Universal Numbering System—permanent dentition (Base art copyright by the American Dental Association. Reprinted by permission.)

Deciduous Teeth

The deciduous teeth are numbered consecutively in the same manner as the permanent teeth from the maxillary right second molar to the maxillary left second molar using the letter "d," for deciduous, with the number of the tooth, Figure 4-2. For example, the deciduous maxillary right second molar is d-1; the mandibular left canine is d-13. Capital letters "A" through "T" can also be used in the same way to designate the deciduous dentition.

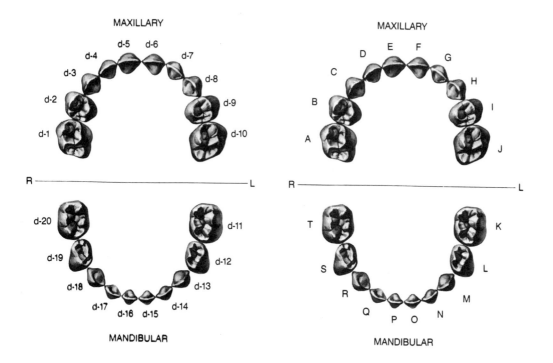

Figure 4-2 Universal Numbering System—decidious dentition
(Base art copyright by the American Dental Association.
Reprinted by permission.)

PALMER'S NOTATION

Palmer's Notation designates each tooth according to its location in a quadrant.
A horizontal line separates the maxilla from the mandible and a vertical midline
separates the patient's right and left sides of the mouth, as shown in Figure 4-3.

Permanent teeth are numbered 1 - 8 in each quadrant beginning at the central incisor to the third molar. Deciduous teeth are designated with the letters A - E.

When identifying an individual tooth, a right angle is used to identify the
quadrant and arch as follows:

maxillary right	maxillary left
mandibular right	mandibular left

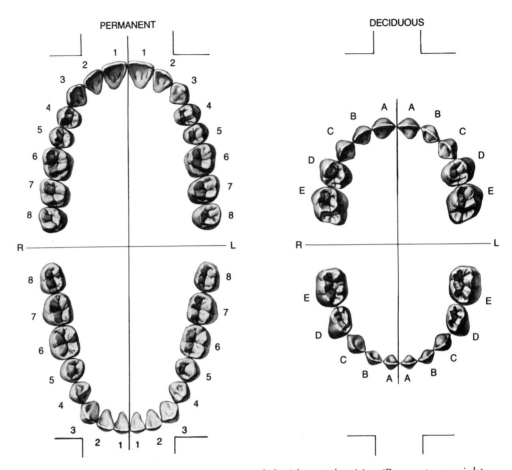

Figure 4-3 Palmer's Notation—permanent and deciduous dentition (Base art copyright by the American Dental Association. Reprinted by permission.)

The tooth number is written within the angle:

Permanent maxillary right central incisor   1⌐

Permanent mandibular left first premolar   ⌐4

Deciduous maxillary left second molar   └E

Deciduous mandibular right canine   C⌐

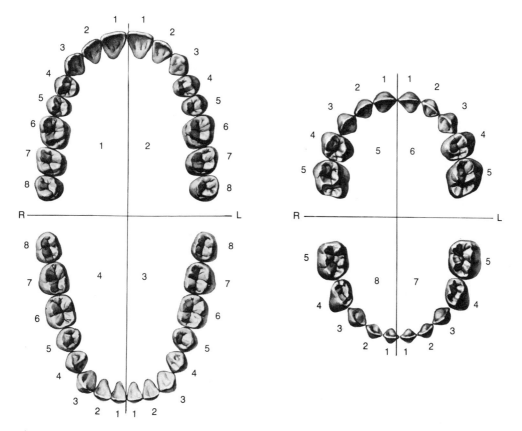

Figure 4-4 Federation Dentaire Internationale (FDI) (Base art copyright by the American Dental Association. Reprinted by permission.)

FEDERATION DENTAIRE INTERNATIONALE (FDI)

The FDI numbering system was introduced to provide a standard international system of coding teeth, Figure 4-4. Each quadrant is assigned a number:

Permanent Teeth

Maxillary right	1
Maxillary left	2
Mandibular left	3
Mandibular right	4

Deciduous Teeth

Maxillary right	5
Maxillary left	6
Mandibular left	7
Mandibular right	8

The teeth within each quadrant are then numbered 1-8, from the central incisor to the third molar, as with Palmer's Notation. The deciduous teeth are numbered 1-5.

To use this system, a two-digit figure identifies each tooth: the first digit designates the dentition, arch, and quadrant; the second digit codes the individual tooth. For example:

Permanent Maxillary right	⟶ 1	3 ◀—	canine		13
Permanent Mandibular left	⟶ 3	1 ◀—	central incisor		31
Deciduous Maxillary left	⟶ 6	4 ◀—	first molar		64
Deciduous Mandibular right	⟶ 8	2 ◀—	lateral incisor		82

SUMMARY

The three numbering systems described: Palmer's Notation, The Universal Numbering System, and the Federation Dentaire Internationale (FDI) are the most commonly used standards for identifying and charting the teeth. Numbering systems provide a basis for coding the conditions of the teeth in a manner that is efficient and convenient for dental personnel.

WORKSHEET

A. Identify the appropriate code for each tooth listed.

	UNIVERSAL NUMBER	PALMER'S NOTATION	FDI
Permanent Teeth			
Maxillary right second molar			
Maxillary left canine			
Maxillary left central incisor			
Mandibular left first premolar			
Mandibular right canine			
Maxillary right lateral incisor			
Mandibular right second molar			
Mandibular left first molar			
Deciduous Teeth			
Mandibular right canine			
Maxillary left second molar			
Mandibular left central incisor			
Maxillary right lateral incisor			
Mandibular left first molar			

SECTION TWO
PERMANENT ANTERIOR TEETH

Introductory Information

INTRODUCTORY INFORMATION

After you have finished this section, you will be able to identify the location in the dental arch of each anterior tooth, as well as its universal number, expected eruption date, usual crown and root completion dates, function, lengths of crown and root, antagonists, and location of contact areas, number of lobes, and pulp canals. You will be able to state at what age there is evidence of calcification in the formation of each tooth.

You will be able to describe the location and/or contour of the incisal edge or cusp slopes, the mesial and distal outlines, contact areas, surface characteristics, the developmental depressions, root shape, cervical lines, and lingual structures.

You will also be able to define terms such as anomaly, cingulum, developmental depression, fossa, groove, lobe, pit, and furrow.

Certain characteristics and structures are common to all anterior teeth. To assist in understanding the tooth morphology, and avoid repetition throughout the chapters, the following related information provides a general background applicable to all anterior teeth.

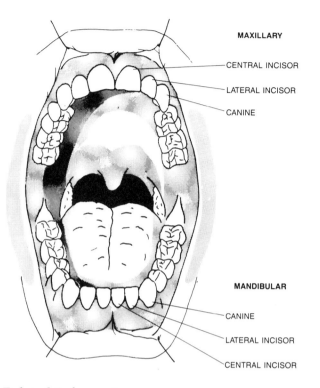

Figure II-1 Permanent anterior teeth (Reprinted, by permission, from Anderson & Burkard, *The Dental Assistant,* Fig. 9–1. © 1982 by Delmar Publishers Inc.)

Related Information

Lobe. A lobe is a center of development and calcification from which a tooth is formed, Figure II-1. All anterior teeth develop from four lobes that eventually coalesce to shape the crown. Three lobes form the labial surface of the crown and the fourth lobe shapes a cingulum on the lingual surface. Demarcations of lobe coalescence are evident as linear depressions on the labial surface.

Mamelons. These make up a scalloped border along the incisal edge of the incisors present at the eruption of the teeth. These are remnants of lobe formation and are worn away by attrition shortly after eruption, Figure II-2.

Cervical Line. The cervical line, or cemento-enamel junction (CEJ) is a demarcation separating the anatomical crown and root. When viewing the tooth from the labial or lingual surface, the cervical line appears as a semi-circle curving toward the root. From the proximal surface, the cervical line curves incisally. Its depth varies from 1-3 mm; this is significant when the teeth are being scaled. For further information on this see Chapter 17.

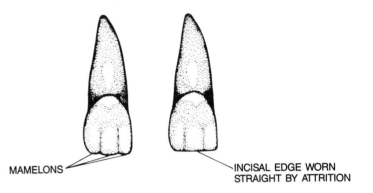

MAMELONS   INCISAL EDGE WORN
                                                  STRAIGHT BY ATTRITION

Figure II-2 Maxillary right central incisor—labial surface

Root Apex. The apex is the tip of the root. In most instances, the root tip of an anterior tooth has a distal inclination. The exception is the mandibular canine which frequently has a mesially inclined root tip.

Pulp Canal. The portion of the pulp that is in the root of the tooth. All anterior teeth have one root and one pulp canal.

Antagonist. A tooth that contacts another tooth in the opposite arch. Mandibular teeth contact maxillary teeth; they are the antagonists of each other. All anterior teeth have two antagonists *except* the mandibular central incisors which have only one, Figure II-3.

Succedaneous Tooth. A permanent tooth that replaces, or succeeds, a deciduous tooth in the same position. Each permanent anterior tooth succeeds a deciduous anterior tooth; i.e., the permanent maxillary central incisor succeeds the deciduous maxillary central incisor. The permanent incisor is the succedaneous tooth.

Structures Common to all Anterior Teeth

Fossa. A shallow rounded depression.

Ridge. A linear elevation. Ridges are named by their location; for example, the mesial marginal ridge or lingual ridge.

Cingulum. A convex, or rounded, elevation or tubercle on the cervical third of the lingual surface. This is a remnant of the fourth, or lingual, lobe.

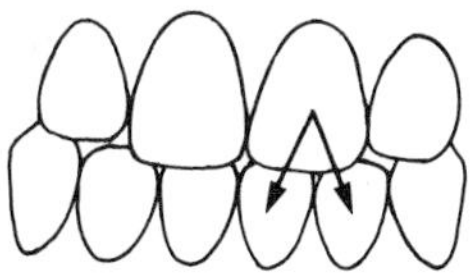

Figure II-3 All anterior teeth have two antagonists except the mandibular central incisor.

Developmental Depression or Furrow. A shallow, linear concavity located on either the crown or root.

Pit. A pinpoint depression.

5

Maxillary Incisors

GENERAL INFORMATION
MAXILLARY CENTRAL INCISOR
MAXILLARY LATERAL INCISOR

Objectives

- Identify the maxillary incisors and provide vital information:
  i.e., universal number, function, antagonist, etc.
- Describe the location and contour of each maxillary incisor.
- Define the new terms in the chapter.
- Complete the worksheet at the end of the chapter.

GENERAL INFORMATION

There are four maxillary incisors: two central and two lateral incisors. Each quadrant has only one central incisor and one lateral incisor. Both the central and lateral incisors are similar in shape; however, the lateral incisor is smaller and slightly more convex. See Figure 5-1 for a comparison of the size of the maxillary central incisor.

At eruption, mamelons are more prominent on the central incisor, but are worn away by attrition after a short period of use. Incisors are wedge-shaped (see Figure 5-8) with a straight, sharp cutting, or incisal, edge that makes them adaptable for incising food.

A frequent deviation of the maxillary central incisor is a variation in root length, the most common of which is a short or blunted root, Figure 5-2.

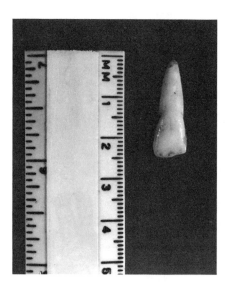

Figure 5-1 Relative size of the maxillary central incisor

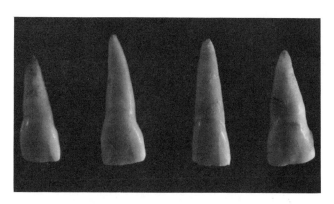

Figure 5-2 Maxillary central incisor—size variation

The maxillary lateral incisor is the tooth, other than third molars, that most commonly forms as an *anomaly.* Its most frequent variation of crown shape is the "peg-shaped" lateral, Figure 5-3.

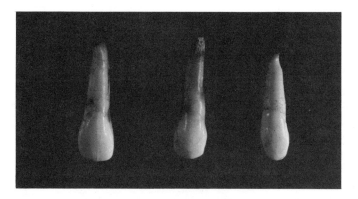

Figure 5-3 Maxillary lateral incisor—normal and two anomalies

MAXILLARY CENTRAL INCISOR

CHARACTERISTICS
    LOCATION IN THE ARCH . . . . .One on either side of midline
    UNIVERSAL NUMBER. . . . . .R-#8   L-#9
    ERUPTION DATE . . . . .7-8 years
    FIRST EVIDENCE OF CALCIFICATION . . . . .3-4 months
    CROWN COMPLETION . . . . .4-5 years
    ROOT COMPLETION . . . . .10 years
    FUNCTION . . . . .biting, incising
    LENGTH OF CROWN. . . . . .10.5 mm
    LENGTH OF ROOT . . . . .13 mm
    ANTAGONISTS. . . . . .Mandibular central and lateral
                                         incisors

LOCATION OF CONTACT AREA
    MESIAL . . . . .Mesio-incisal angle
    DISTAL . . . . .Slightly cervical to disto-incisal
                                         angle

IDENTIFYING FEATURES
    • widest anterior tooth mesio-distally
    • straight mesial side with sharp mesio-incisal angle and convex distal side
    • straight incisal edge
    • wedge shape of tooth

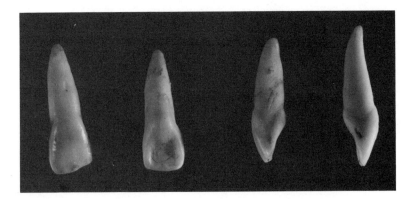

Figure 5-4 Maxillary central incisor

Tooth Description of the Maxillary Central Incisor

Labial Surface. After the mamelons are worn away, the incisal edge is straight, slightly inclining toward the distal side of the tooth. The mesio-incisal angle is sharp, contacting the mesial of the adjacent central incisor at the incisal edge. Tapering gradually, the mesial side continues straight until it merges with the cervical line, Figure 5-5. The disto-incisal angle, slightly rounded, forms the distal contact area just cervical to the incisal edge. The distal side of the tooth is slightly convex, tapering until it joins the cervical line, a semicircle. Two slight vertical developmental depressions, the result of lobe formation, are present on the labial surface; otherwise it is smooth. A cone-shaped root tapers gradually to a blunt apex.

Lingual Surface. The outline of the lingual surface is the reverse of the labial view. A well-defined lingual fossa is outlined by marginal ridges and the cingulum, Figure 5-6. Frequently, shallow grooves are found in the fossa. A pronounced cingulum dominates the cervical third of the crown.

Proximal Surfaces. Seen from this view is a typical wedge-shape that renders the tooth adaptable for biting and incising food. Note that the cervical line curves incisally for about one third the length of the crown, Figure 5-7.

The root is broad and smooth (no depressions or furrows) and tapers, in the apical third, to a blunt apex. The tip of the root and the incisal edge are on the midline providing balance for the tooth when functioning.

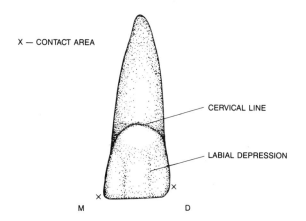

X — CONTACT AREA

CERVICAL LINE

LABIAL DEPRESSION

M   D

Figure 5-5 Maxillary left central incisor—labial surface

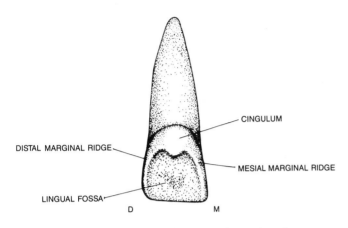

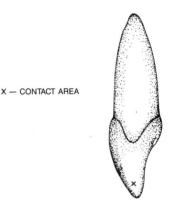

Figure 5-6 Maxillary central incisor—lingual surface

Figure 5-7 Maxillary central incisor—proximal surface

Summary of the Maxillary Central Incisor

Labial Surface. The characteristics of this surface are:

- A straight incisal edge, inclining toward distal
- A straight mesial side
- A sharp mesio-incisal angle
- A mesial contact area (X) located at the mesio-incisal angle
- A slightly convex distal side
- A rounded disto-incisal angle
- A distal contact area (X) located in the incisal third
- Developmental depressions on the crown
- A cone shaped root with a blunt apex

Lingual Surface. The characteristics of this surface are:

- An outline that is the reverse of the labial
- A concave lingual fossa
- Mesial and distal marginal ridges that outline the fossa
- A convex cingulum that makes up the cervical third of the crown

Proximal Surfaces. The characteristics of these surfaces are:

- A cervical line that curves one third of the tooth toward the incisal
- The tip of the incisal edge and the root are on the midline
- A root that is broad and tapers in the apical third
- There are no furrows or depressions on the root

MAXILLARY LATERAL INCISOR

CHARACTERISTICS
LOCATION IN THE ARCH . . . . Distal to central incisor; second
tooth from midline
UNIVERSAL NUMBER . . . . R-#7 L-#10
ERUPTION DATE . . . . 8-9 years
FIRST EVIDENCE OF CALCIFICATION . . . . 1 year
CROWN COMPLETION . . . . 4-5 years
ROOT COMPLETION . . . . 11 years
FUNCTION . . . . biting, incising
LENGTH OF CROWN . . . . 9 mm
LENGTH OF ROOT . . . . 13 mm
ANTAGONISTS . . . . Mandibular lateral incisor and
canine

LOCATION OF CONTACT AREA
MESIAL . . . . Junction of middle and incisal third
DISTAL . . . . Middle third

IDENTIFYING FEATURES
- resembles maxillary central incisor but is smaller with more convex mesial and distal sides and incisal angles
- developmental variations are frequent

(Refer to Figure 5-8 on page 54.)

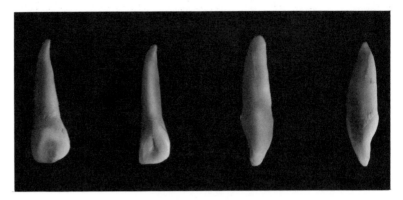

Figure 5-8 Maxillary lateral incisor

Tooth Description of the Maxillary Lateral Incisor

Labial Surface. The lateral incisor has the same shape as the central incisor but is smaller and slightly more convex, Figure 5-9. The incisal edge inclines toward the distal. Both the mesial and distal incisal angles are rounded and both the mesial and distal sides of the tooth are convex. Although developmental depressions may be present, the labial surface is usually smooth. Both mesial and distal contact areas are located more cervically than on the central incisor. A cone-shaped root tapers, gradually, toward the apex.

Lingual Surface. The lingual outline is the reverse of the labial, Figure 5-10. However, the cingulum is very pronounced with a developmental pit located in

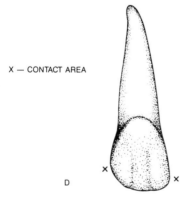

X — CONTACT AREA

D   X   X   M

Figure 5-9 Maxillary right lateral incisor—labial surface

CINGULUM —   — LINGUAL PIT

— DISTAL MARGINAL RIDGE

MESIAL MARGINAL RIDGE —   — LINGUAL FOSSA

Figure 5-10 Maxillary right lateral incisor—lingual surface

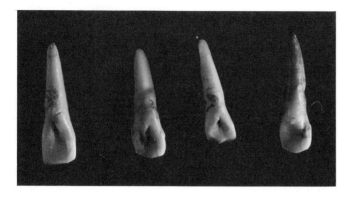

Figure 5-11 Maxillary lateral incisor—lingual pit

the fossa directly beneath it, Figure 5-11. The lingual fossa is more likely to have developmental grooves than the maxillary central incisor. All other structures are the same as the central incisor.

Proximal Surfaces. The structures and shape, from this view, are the same as the maxillary central incisor. However, there is a furrow, or long, shallow depression, present on the root, Figure 5-12.

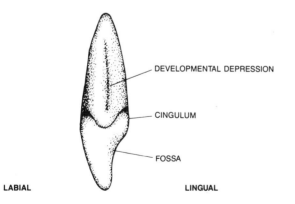

Figure 5-12 Maxillary lateral incisor—proximal surface

Summary of the Maxillary Lateral Incisor

Labial Surface. The characteristics of this surface are:

- A straight incisal edge that inclines toward the distal.
- Rounded mesial and distal incisal angles.
- Convex mesial and distal sides.
- Mesial and distal contact areas that are more cervical than the central incisor.
- A smooth labial surface.
- A tapered root.

Lingual Surface. The characteristics of this surface are:

- A prominent cingulum.
- A developmental pit that is in the fossa below the cingulum.

Proximal Surface. The characteristics of this surface are:

- A wedge-shape outline that is the same as the maxillary central incisor.
- A cervical line that curves one third of the tooth toward the incisal.
- A root that is broad with furrows on both the mesial and distal surfaces.

SUMMARY

Incisors are wedge-shaped teeth with sharp, straight incisal edges used to cut or incise food. Both the maxillary central and lateral incisors have similar shapes, although the lateral incisor is smaller and slightly more convex.

WORKSHEET

A. Complete the chart with the information requested.

	CENTRAL INCISOR	LATERAL INCISOR
Universal Number		
Palmer's Notation		
Eruption Date		
Antagonists		
Location of Contact		
Mesial		
Distal		
Succedaneous		
Number of Lobes		
Labial Depressions*		
Lingual*		
Ridges		
Cingulum		
Fossa		
Root Shape		
Labial		
Proximal		

*Indicate location, size, and/or shape

B. Use the following figure to complete the questions.

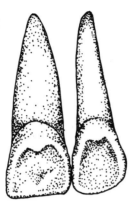

1. Draw and label the cingulum, mesial and distal marginal ridges, and fossa.

2. Place an "X" at both mesial and distal contact areas.

3. What structure is present on the maxillary lateral, lingual surface that is not included on the central incisor, lingual?

C. Use the following figure to complete the questions.

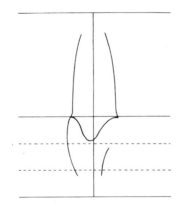

1. Draw in the root tip and the incisal edge.

2. Draw the cingulum.

6
Mandibular Incisors

GENERAL INFORMATION
MANDIBULAR CENTRAL INCISOR
MANDIBULAR LATERAL INCISOR

Objectives

- Identify the mandibular incisors and provide vital information: i.e., universal number, function, antagonist, etc.
- Describe the location and contour of each mandibular incisor.
- Define the new terms in the chapter.
- Complete the worksheet at the end of the chapter.

GENERAL INFORMATION

There are four mandibular incisors: two central incisors and two lateral incisors. Each quadrant has one central and one lateral incisor.

The central and lateral incisors appear quite similar although the lateral incisor is larger. The opposite situation exists in the maxilla where the central is larger than the lateral incisor.

As the smallest tooth in the dentition, the mandibular central incisor has only one antagonist, Figure 6-1. This tooth and the maxillary third molar are the only teeth that have one antagonist; all others have two antagonists.

Shortly after eruption, mamelons are worn away by attrition and the incisal edges of all incisors are straight. Viewed from the proximal surface, the mandibular incisors have the same wedge-shape as the maxillary incisors, and so are suited for incising food.

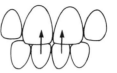

Figure 6-1 The mandibular central incisor has only one antagonist.

MANDIBULAR CENTRAL INCISOR

CHARACTERISTICS

    LOCATION IN THE ARCH . . . . .One, on either side of the midline

    UNIVERSAL NUMBER. . . . . .R-#25   L-#24

    ERUPTION DATE . . . . .6-7 years

    FIRST EVIDENCE OF CALCIFICATION . . . . .3-4 months

    CROWN COMPLETION . . . . .4-5 years

    ROOT COMPLETION . . . . .9 years

    FUNCTION . . . . .Incising, biting

    LENGTH OF CROWN. . . . . .9 mm

    LENGTH OF ROOT . . . . .12.5 mm

    ANTAGONIST. . . . . .Maxillary central incisor

LOCATION OF CONTACT AREA

    MESIAL . . . . .Mesial incisal angle

    DISTAL . . . . .Distal incisal angle

IDENTIFYING FEATURES

    • smallest tooth in the oral cavity

    • bilaterally symmetrical from labial or lingual view

    • smooth tooth; no developmental grooves or depression in crown

    • only one antagonist

(Refer to Figure 6-2.)

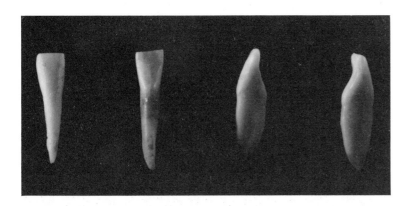

Figure 6-2 Mandibular central incisor

Tooth Description of the Mandibular Central Incisor

Labial Surface. The incisal edge is straight joining the mesial and distal sides at sharp incisal angles, Figure 6-3. These angles are the contact areas. Both mesial and distal sides are straight, tapering evenly to the cervix where the cervical line forms an arc.

The tooth is bilaterally symmetrical — the same on both sides — so it is difficult to differentiate the mesial from the distal side. The root is straight, tapering gradually to the apex.

Lingual Surface. The outline from the lingual is the reverse of the labial view. This surface is very smooth; there are no pits or grooves and the fossa and cingulum merge with a gentle curve, Figure 6-4. Marginal ridges are not evident

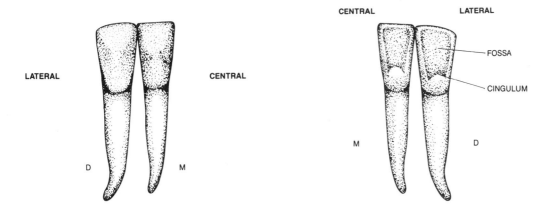

Figure 6-3 Mandibular right incisor—labial view

Figure 6-4 Mandibular right incisor—lingual surface

as was seen on the maxillary incisors. The cingulum covers the cervical third of the crown; the fossa occupies the remaining two thirds.

Proximal Surfaces. The width, from labial to lingual, is broad to compensate for the narrow mesial to distal measurements seen from the labial view. The width is necessary to provide stability for such a small tooth. The root remains broad for two thirds its length, tapering only at the apical third. Both the mesial and distal root surfaces have a deep depression extending most of the root length, Figure 6-5.

The incisal edge of the mandibular incisor is positioned lingual to the midline. When the teeth occlude, the labial surface of the mandibular incisors conform to the lingual fossa of the maxillary incisors, Figure 6-6.

Incisal View. Observing this tooth from the incisal aspect assists in differentiating it from the mandibular lateral incisor. The central incisor has a straight incisal edge that is bilaterally symmetrical, Figure 6-7. Usually, it is difficult to distinguish the mesial side from the distal side of the crown because of their similarity in structure.

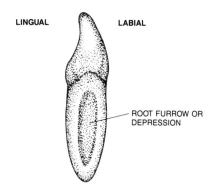

LINGUAL   LABIAL

ROOT FURROW OR DEPRESSION

Figure 6-5 Mandibular right incisor—proximal surface

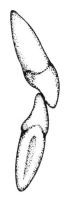

Figure 6-6 Incisors in occlusion—proximal view

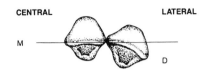

Figure 6-7 Mandibular incisor—
incisal view

Summary of the Mandibular Central Incisor

Labial Surface. The characteristics of this surface are:

- A straight incisal edge with sharp incisal angles.
- Mesial and distal sides that taper evenly to the cervix.
- Mesial and distal contact areas that are located at the incisal angle.
- A smooth crown surface with no depressions.
- A straight root, tapering at the apical third.

Lingual Surface. The characteristics of this surface are:

- An outline that is the reverse of the labial view.
- A smooth fossa; a smooth cingulum.
- A convex cingulum that is one third of the crown.

Proximal Surfaces. The characteristics of these surfaces are:

- The tip of the incisal edge sitting lingual to the midline.
- A cervical line that curves toward the incisal edge.
- A broad root, tapering at the apical third.
- A root furrow or depression on the mesial and distal surfaces.

Incisal View. The characteristics of this surface are:

- A straight incisal ridge.
- A bilaterally symmetrical form.

MANDIBULAR LATERAL INCISOR

CHARACTERISTICS
  LOCATION IN THE ARCH . . . . .Distal to central incisor; second tooth
                                                                    from midline
  UNIVERSAL NUMBER. . . . . .R-#26   L-#23
  ERUPTION DATE . . . . .7-8 years
  FIRST EVIDENCE OF CALCIFICATION . . . . .3-4 months
  CROWN COMPLETION . . . . .4-5 years
  ROOT COMPLETION . . . . .10 years
  FUNCTION . . . . .Biting, incising
  LENGTH OF CROWN. . . . . .9.5 mm
  LENGTH OF ROOT . . . . .14 mm
  ANTAGONISTS. . . . . .Maxillary central and lateral incisors

LOCATION OF CONTACT AREA
  MESIAL . . . . .Mesial incisal angle
  DISTAL . . . . .Cervical to the incisal angle

IDENTIFYING FEATURES
  • slightly larger than the central incisor
  • slightly more convex than the central incisor
  • incisal ridge curves to the distal

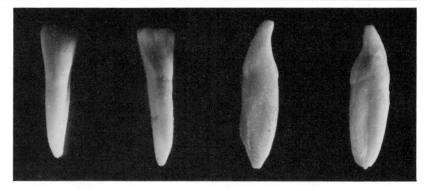

Figure 6-8 Mandibular lateral incisor

Tooth Description of the Mandibular Lateral Incisor

Labial Surface. The lateral incisor looks like the central incisor in overall appearance but is slightly larger and not bilaterally symmetrical (see Figure 6-3). Whereas the central incisor has a level incisal edge, the incisal edge of the lateral declines toward the distal and forms a rounded incisal angle with the distal side. The distal side is slightly convex. The mesial incisal angle is sharp; the mesial side can be straight or slightly convex as it tapers toward the cervical line. Both the mesial and distal contact areas are at the incisal angle. The cervical line forms a narrow arch. The root is straight, tapering at the apical third.

Lingual and Proximal Surfaces. Except for size and length, the mandibular lateral incisor is similar to the central incisor and has the same characteristics (see Figure 6-4).

Incisal View. The incisal edge of the lateral incisor curves toward the distal, following the contour of the mandibular arch, whereas the incisal edge of the central incisor is straight. The curvature on the lateral incisor creates a distally displaced cingulum as compared to the centrally situated cingulum of the central incisor. This structure assists in distinguishing the two teeth from each other, see Figure 6-9.

Summary of the Mandibular Lateral Incisor

Labial Surface. The characteristics of this surface are:

- An incisal edge that declines toward the distal.
- A mesial surface that tapers gradually toward the cervix.

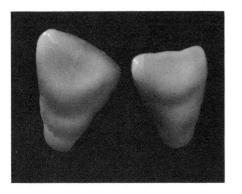

Figure 6-9 Mandibular central and lateral incisor—incisal view

- A distal side that is slightly convex, tapering toward the cervix.
- A sharp mesial incisal angle; a rounded distal incisal angle.
- Mesial and distal contact areas that are at the junction of the incisal edge and the mesial or distal side.
- A smooth surface.
- A straight root that tapers evenly.

Lingual Surface. The characteristics of this surface are:

- An outline that is the reverse of the labial side.
- Other structures that are the same as the central incisor.

Proximal Surfaces. The characteristics of these surfaces are:

- Root depressions on the mesial and distal sides; the distal depression is deeper.
- Characteristics that are all the same as the central incisor.

Incisal View. The characteristics of this view are:

- An incisal edge that curves toward the distal.
- A cingulum that is distally displaced.

SUMMARY

Mandibular incisors assist the maxillary incisors in biting and cutting food. From the labial view, both mandibular incisors are small, narrow teeth with a straight incisal edge, tapering along both the mesial and distal sides. The mandibular central incisor is the smallest tooth in the dentition.

WORKSHEET

A. Complete the chart with the information requested.

	CENTRAL INCISOR	LATERAL INCISOR
Universal Number		
Palmer's Notation		
Eruption Date		
Antagonists		
Location of Contact		
Mesial		
Distal		
Succedaneous		
Number of Lobes		
Labial Depressions*		
Lingual*		
Ridges		
Cingulum		
Fossa		
Root Shape		
Labial		
Proximal		

*Indicate location, size, and/or shape

B. Complete the following questions.

1. The figure below shows the labial surface of the mandibular central and lateral incisors. Complete the drawing by adding the incisal, mesial, and distal surfaces of each.

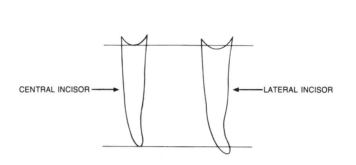

2. The figure below shows an outline of the incisal view of the mandibular central incisor. Draw the incisal edge. Draw the mandibular lateral incisor, incisal view, in contact with the central incisor.

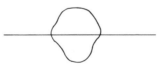

3. This figure shows the proximal surface of a mandibular incisor. Complete the drawing to show the correct relationship of the incisal edge to the root tip.

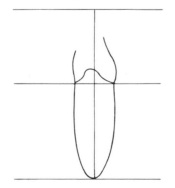

7

Canines

GENERAL INFORMATION
MAXILLARY CANINE
MANDIBULAR CANINE

Objectives

- Identify the canines and provide vital information: i.e., universal number, function, antagonist, etc.
- Describe the location and contour of each canine.
- Define the new terms in the chapter.
- Complete the worksheet at the end of the chapter.

GENERAL INFORMATION

There are two canines in each arch: one in each quadrant. Maxillary and mandibular canines look like each other, showing only minor variations as noted in the descriptions. Both canines have a sharp, pointed cusp, thus attaining their alternate name of "cuspids." They are long, strong, stable teeth. Note their size and length (Figure 7-1) as compared to their adjacent teeth.

Because they are located at the corner of each arch, canines are referred to as the "cornerstone" teeth. Their position is important to aesthetics because they provide shape to the face. If dentures are needed and the size or position of the canine is varied, the entire facial appearance can change. Fortunately, canines are self-cleansing, because of their convexity and location at the corners of the arch, so that food easily rolls off them. Thus, they are usually the last teeth to be lost due to dental decay. The shape of this tooth, particularly the sharp cusp, makes it adaptable for holding and tearing food.

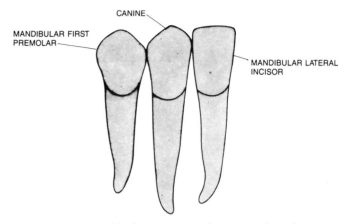

Figure 7-1 Mandibular canine with proximal teeth

MAXILLARY CANINE

CHARACTERISTICS
LOCATION IN THE ARCH . . . . Distal to lateral incisor; third tooth from midline

UNIVERSAL NUMBER. . . . . R-#6   L-#11
ERUPTION DATE . . . . 11-12 years
FIRST EVIDENCE OF CALCIFICATION . . . . 4-5 months
CROWN COMPLETION . . . . 6-7 years
ROOT COMPLETION . . . . 13-15 years
FUNCTION . . . . Tearing, holding
LENGTH OF CROWN. . . . . 10 mm
LENGTH OF ROOT. . . . . 17 mm
ANTAGONIST. . . . . Mandibular canine and first premolar

LOCATION OF CONTACT AREA
MESIAL . . . . Junction of incisal and middle third
DISTAL . . . . Middle third

(Chart continued on the following page)

IDENTIFYING FEATURES
- longest maxillary tooth
- stable, sturdy tooth
- cornerstone of the arch
- sharp, pointed cusp
- bulky cingulum and defined lingual ridges

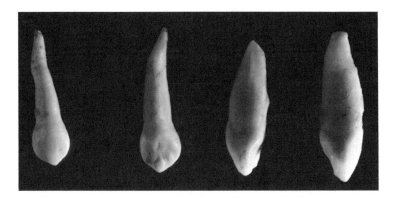

Figure 7-2 Maxillary canine

Tooth Description of the Maxillary Canine

Labial Surface. From the tip of the cusp to both the mesial and distal contact areas is a cusp slope rather than an incisal edge that is seen on the incisors. Both contact areas are located near the junction of the incisal and middle third of the tooth, noted with an "X" on Figure 7-3. The mesial cusp slope is shorter than the distal cusp slope. It joins the mesial surface at the junction of the incisal and middle third; the mesial side is convex. Because of a longer cusp slope, the distal contact area is more cervical than the mesial and located in the middle third of the crown. The distal side of the tooth is slightly concave before merging with the cervical line.

A well-developed middle lobe, called the labial ridge, is centrally located and extends from the cervix to the tip of the cusp. Shallow depressions extend, vertically, along both sides of the ridge. The root is cone-shaped and usually smooth.

Lingual Surface. The outline is the reverse of the labial view, but narrower. Forming the lingual surface are the fossae and a well-pronounced cingulum, Figure 7-4. The cingulum is situated in the cervical third of the crown. A lingual ridge divides the fossa into two segments, a mesial fossa and distal fossa. This lingual ridge extends from the base of the cingulum to the cusp tip. Raised mesial and distal marginal ridges outline the lateral border of the fossae.

Proximal Surfaces. Both the length and width of this canine, as seen from either proximal surface, are greater than other anterior teeth, Figure 7-5. The width is needed to give the tooth stability. The root is broad for two thirds its length, tapering only at the apical third. Deep depressions on the mesial and distal root give the tooth the greater stability needed during mastication.

Summary of the Maxillary Canine

Labial Surface. The characteristics of this surface are:

- A mesial cusp slope that is shorter than the distal cusp slope.
- A mesial contact area that is at the junction of the incisal and the middle third.
- A distal contact area that is in the middle third of the tooth.
- A slightly convex mesial side.

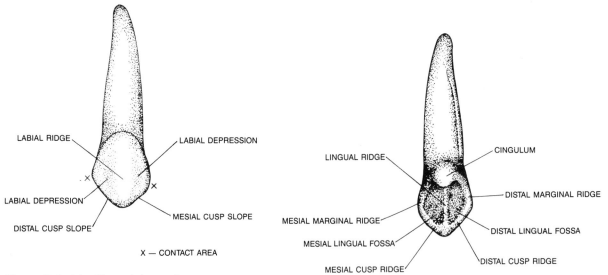

Figure 7-3 Maxillary right canine—labial surface

Figure 7-4 Maxillary right canine—lingual surface

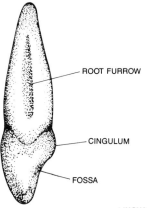

ROOT FURROW

CINGULUM

FOSSA

LABIAL   LINGUAL   **Figure 7-5** Maxillary canine—proximal surface

- A slightly concave distal side.
- A well-developed middle lobe, called the labial ridge.
- Depressions that are on either side of the labial ridge.
- A cusp tip that is centered over the root.
- A cone-shaped, smooth root.

Lingual Surface. The characteristics of this surface are:

- An outline that is the reverse of the labial view.
- A crown and root that converge so that both mesial and distal surfaces can be seen.
- A fossa that is divided, by a lingual ridge, into a mesio-lingual and disto-lingual fossa.
- A pronounced cingulum and marginal ridges.

Proximal Surfaces. The characteristics of these surfaces are:

- A broad crown and root.
- A cervical line that curves toward the incisal.
- A deep depression in the root surface.

MANDIBULAR CANINE

CHARACTERISTICS

    LOCATION IN THE ARCH . . . . Distal to lateral incisor; third tooth
                                                           from midline

    UNIVERSAL NUMBER . . . . R-#27   L-#22

    ERUPTION DATE . . . . 9-10 years

    FIRST EVIDENCE OF CALCIFICATION . . . . 4-5 months

    CROWN COMPLETION . . . . 6-7 years

    ROOT COMPLETION . . . . 12-14 years

    FUNCTION . . . . Tearing, holding

    LENGTH OF CROWN . . . . 11 mm

    LENGTH OF ROOT . . . . 16 mm

    ANTAGONISTS . . . . Maxillary lateral incisor and canine

LOCATION OF CONTACT AREA

    MESIAL . . . . Incisal third

    DISTAL . . . . Junction of incisal and middle third

IDENTIFYING FEATURES

- longest mandibular tooth
- well-developed middle lobe called labial ridge
- slightly narrower and smoother than maxillary canine

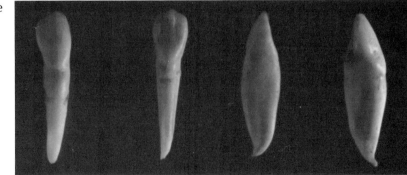

Figure 7-6 Mandibular canine

Tooth Description of the Mandibular Canine

Labial Surface. The mandibular canine looks like the maxillary canine but is narrower by 0.5 mm. It appears even narrower than this, as compared to the maxillary canine, because both the mesial and distal contact areas are located more incisally.

The mesial cusp slope is shorter than the distal; the mesial side of the tooth is straight and the distal side is slightly more convex, Figure 7-7. The labial ridge is not as prominent as on the maxillary canine.

Lingual Surface. The outline is the reverse of the labial view, but narrower. The structures are the same as those on the maxillary canine, but less pronounced, Figure 7-8.

Proximal Surfaces. Again, the tooth is broad from this view with an overall shape resembling the maxillary canine, Figure 7-9.

Summary of the Mandibular Canine

Labial Surface. The characteristics of this surface are:

- A mesial cusp slope that is shorter than the distal.
- Contact areas that are more incisal than on the maxillary canine.
- A straight mesial side.
- A slightly convex distal side.
- A tapered root

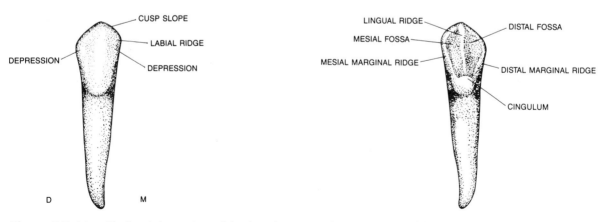

Figure 7-7 Mandibular right canine—labial surface   **Figure 7-8** Mandibular right canine—lingual surface

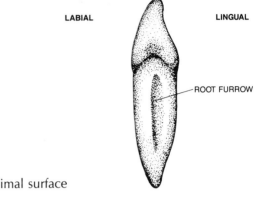

Figure 7-9 Mandibular canine—proximal surface

Lingual Surface. The characteristics of this surface are:

- An outline that is the reverse of the labial view, but narrower.
- Cingulum and marginal ridges that are smoother than the maxillary canine.
- Two fossae that are divided by the lingual ridge.
- A fossa that is shallower than on the maxillary canine.

Proximal Surfaces. The characteristics of these surfaces are:

- Greater width, providing stability.
- Deep depressions on the root surface.

SUMMARY

Canines, along with the incisors, are considered anterior teeth. Both maxillary and mandibular canines are broad, pointed teeth with a sharp cusp that is used to tear food when necessary. These strong, stable teeth are located at the corners of the arch, thus providing shape to the face.

WORKSHEET

A. Complete the chart with the information requested.

	MAXILLARY	MANDIBULAR
Universal Number		
Palmer's Notation		
Eruption Date		
Antagonists		
Location of Contact		
Mesial		
Distal		
Succedaneous		
Number of Lobes		
*Labial Depressions**		
*Lingual**		
Ridges		
Cingulum		
Fossa		
Root Shape		
Labial		
Proximal		

*Indicate location, size, and/or shape

B. Using the figure below, complete the following information.

MANDIBULAR   MAXILLARY

1. Which of the two canines is larger? _____

2. Which tooth in the permanent dentition is longer? _____

3. Compare the contact areas. On which tooth are they more incisal? _____

4. Label the cusp slopes. Is the mesial or the distal cusp slope shorter? _____

5. Draw the following structures on the maxillary canine:
   Cingulum
   Mesial marginal ridge
   Distal marginal ridge
   Lingual ridge

6. Label the ridges and fossae on the completed drawing in number 5.

INTRODUCTORY INFORMATION

After you have finished this section, you will be able to identify the location in the dental arch of each posterior tooth, as well as its universal number, expected eruption date, usual crown and root completion dates, function, lengths of crown and root, antagonists and the location of contact areas, number of lobes, and pulp canals. You will be able to state at what age there is evidence of calcification in the formation of each tooth.

You will be able to describe the location and contour of the buccal, lingual, proximal, and occlusal surfaces as they apply to each posterior tooth. Your descriptions will include contact areas, grooves, cusps, pits, ridges, fossae, outlines, contact areas, and roots of the teeth.

You will also be able to define terms such as comminution, interdigitate, bifurcation, and oblique, transverse, and triangular ridges.

To avoid redundancy in each chapter, the following descriptions consolidate information relating to posterior teeth, Figure III-1.

Related Information

Occlusal Surface. This is the chewing surface. All posterior teeth have a chewing surface shaped by cusps, fossae, ridges, and grooves. The cusps of the maxillary teeth sit in the fossae of the mandibular teeth and vice-versa, Figure III-2. Cusps slope toward the grooves so that the teeth interdigitate when in contact with each other.

Lobes. These are the centers of calcification. All teeth develop from at least four lobes. The premolars, with two cusps, develop from four lobes: three buccal and one lingual. The mandibular second premolar, which has three cusps, develops from five lobes: three buccal and two lingual. Lobe formation of molars is equal to the number of cusps on the tooth. If a molar has four cusps, it develops from four lobes.

Figure III-1 Permanent posterior teeth (Reprinted, by permission, from Anderson & Burkard, *The Dental Assistant,* Fig. 9–1. © 1982 by Delmar Publishers Inc.)

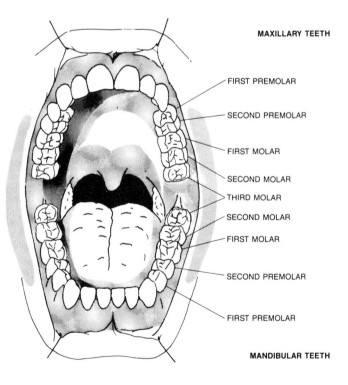

MAXILLARY TEETH

FIRST PREMOLAR

SECOND PREMOLAR

FIRST MOLAR

SECOND MOLAR

THIRD MOLAR

SECOND MOLAR

FIRST MOLAR

SECOND PREMOLAR

FIRST PREMOLAR

MANDIBULAR TEETH

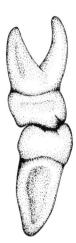

Figure III-2 Molars in occlusion—proximal view

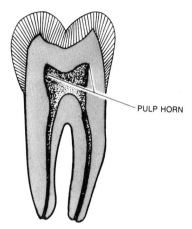

Figure III-3 Pulp horn

Pulp Canals. These are the portions of the pulp located in the root of the tooth. Each root has one pulp canal *except* the mandibular first molar; the mesial root of this tooth has two pulp canals.

Pulp Horn. This is the portion of the pulp chamber, or coronal pulp, that is elevated toward a cusp, Figure III-3.

Root Trunk. This is the portion of the root that extends from the cemento-enamel junction to the furcation. If the root divides into two portions, it is *bifurcated.* All mandibular molars have bifurcated roots. All maxillary molars are *trifurcated* or are divided into three roots. The area on the root trunk where it separates is called the *furcation* or forking, Figure III-4.

MANDIBULAR MOLAR   MAXILLARY MOLAR

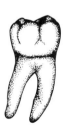

Figure III-4 Furcated roots   BIFURCATED ROOT   TRIFURCATED ROOT

Contact Area. This is the portion of the mesial or distal surface that touches, or contacts, the proximal tooth.

Succedaneous Tooth. This is a tooth that succeeds another tooth in the same position. Premolars are the only posterior teeth that are succedaneous. They succeed the deciduous molars. Permanent molars do not replace deciduous teeth.

Structures Common to all Posterior Teeth

Ridge. A linear elevation, named by its location or direction, Figure III-5. There are several types:

Marginal ridge: The ridges around the perimeter of the occlusal surface.

Transverse ridge: A ridge that crosses the occlusal surface.

Triangular ridge: A ridge that slants from the cusp tip toward a groove and forms a triangular slope.

Oblique ridge: A ridge that crosses the occlusal surface diagonally.

Cusp ridge: A ridge that slopes from the tip of the cusp toward the mesial or distal surface.

Fossae. A shallow depression named by its shape:

Circular fossa: A rounded depression.

Triangular fossa: A "V" shaped depression.

Irregular fossa: A depression without definite shape.

Groove. A linear depression, Figures III-6 and III-7. Each posterior tooth has a primary groove pattern common to that tooth. These groove patterns are

Figure III-5 Maxillary first molar—occlusal view

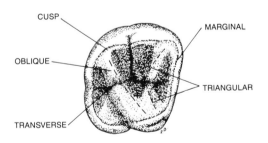

RIDGES

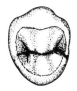
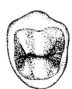

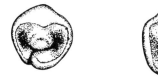

Figure III-6 Review of the groove patterns of the premolars

described in later chapters. Posterior teeth usually have additional or supplementary grooves that are not included with the descriptions or in the illustrations because of their variation in each person.

Pit. A pinpoint depression.

Facts to help avoid confusion

Premolars. Since these teeth usually have two cusps, they are alternately referred to as bicuspids. However, the mandibular second premolar often has three cusps; therefore, these teeth are more accurately called premolars. All premolars have a well-developed middle buccal lobe that forms a buccal ridge, ending at a pointed cusp.

Nomenclature. Cusps, grooves, fossae, and ridges are commonly named by their location, such as mesio-buccal cusp, central groove, or distal marginal ridge. With a little thought, you can probably name most of the structures without having to memorize them. Note that when the words mesial or distal are used in combination with another surface, the "al" is changed to "o" and a hyphen is added, such as "mesio-lingual."

Size and shape of surfaces. Because the mouth has less space toward the posterior region, distal surfaces of the teeth are generally smaller than mesial structures. Crowns, also, tip distally so that more of the occlusal surface can be seen when viewing the distal side of the tooth.

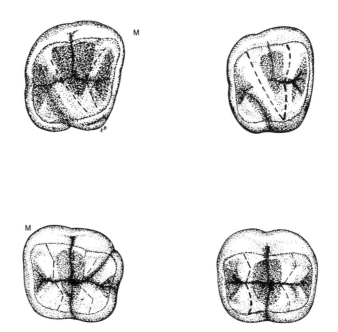

Figure III-7 Review of the groove patterns of the molars

Occlusal surface. Technically, the occlusal surface is within the borders of the marginal ridges. However, when the occlusal surface is described in the following chapters, all structures, seen from this view, are noted.

8

Maxillary Premolars

GENERAL INFORMATION
MAXILLARY FIRST PREMOLAR
MAXILLARY SECOND PREMOLAR

Objectives

- Identify the maxillary premolars and provide vital information: i.e., universal number, function, antagonists, etc.
- Describe the location and contour of each maxillary premolar.
- Define the new terms in the chapter.
- Complete the worksheet at the end of the chapter.

GENERAL INFORMATION

There are four maxillary premolars: two in each quadrant. They are named by their position in the arch from anterior to posterior as first premolar and second premolar.

Maxillary premolars have one buccal and one lingual cusp. Both premolars have a prominent middle buccal lobe extending from the cervix to the tip of the buccal cusp, similar to the canine, with shallow depressions on either side.

The root trunk of the maxillary first premolar is *bifurcated*, dividing into two roots (buccal and lingual) that are seen only from the proximal view. The maxillary second premolar has only one root.

Viewed from the buccal, all premolars resemble each other, with their pointed buccal cusp and tapered root, so that it is difficult to differentiate them. However, each has a unique structure on another surface that will assist in its identification.

Premolars replace deciduous molars; there are no deciduous premolars. The first premolar succeeds the deciduous first molar; the second premolar succeeds the deciduous second molar.

With their triangular-shaped cusps and fossae, the premolars are structured to assist with the grinding of food.

MAXILLARY FIRST PREMOLAR

CHARACTERISTICS
LOCATION IN THE ARCH . . . . Fourth tooth from the midline;
distal to cuspid
UNIVERSAL NUMBER . . . . R-#5   L-#12
ERUPTION DATE . . . . 10-11 years
FIRST EVIDENCE OF CALCIFICATION . . . . 1½ years
CROWN COMPLETION . . . . 5-6 years
ROOT COMPLETION . . . . 12-13 years
FUNCTION . . . . Grinding
LENGTH OF CROWN . . . . 8.5 mm
LENGTH OF ROOT . . . . 14 mm
ANTAGONISTS . . . . Mandibular first and second
premolar

LOCATION OF CONTACT AREA
MESIAL . . . . Middle of the tooth
DISTAL . . . . Slightly more occlusal than the
mesial contact

IDENTIFYING FEATURES
- two cusps: one buccal, one lingual
- two roots: one buccal, one lingual
- two pulp canals: one in each root
- resembles canine but is shorter
- mesial marginal groove

(Refer to Figure 8-1.)

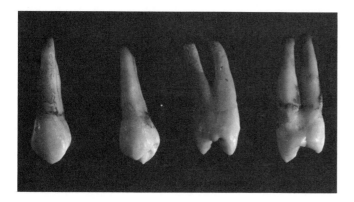

Figure 8-1 Maxillary first premolar

Tooth Description of the Maxillary First Premolar

Buccal Surface. Only the buccal cusp and buccal root are visible, obscuring the shorter lingual cusp and root positioned directly behind them. A well-developed middle buccal lobe forms a buccal ridge extending from the cervix to the tip of the pointed buccal cusp, Figure 8-2. Shallow depressions parallel the ridge. The mesial cusp slope is longer than the distal cusp slope.

The *mesial side* is concave from the cervix to the contact area at the middle of the surface. The *distal side* is straighter than the mesial from the cervix to the contact area. The distal contact area is slightly more occlusal than the mesial, making the distal cusp slope shorter. The buccal root is tapered.

Lingual Surface. Both cusps are visible from this view, Figure 8-3. Since the lingual cusp is 1 mm shorter, the tip of the buccal cusp extends below it. The lingual cusp is smooth — no ridge, no depressions. Some of the mesial and distal surfaces

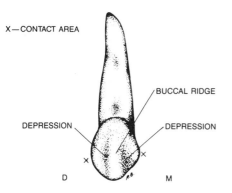

X—CONTACT AREA

BUCCAL RIDGE

DEPRESSION   DEPRESSION

D   M

Figure 8-2 Maxillary right first premolar—buccal surface

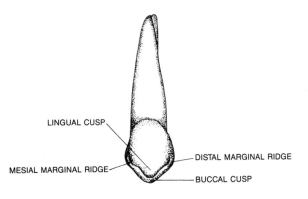

Figure 8-3 Maxillary first premolar—lingual surface

of both the crown and the root are seen because the lingual surface is narrower than the buccal.

Proximal Surfaces. Both cusps and both roots are visible. Although the tooth appears small from the buccal view, it is wider by 2 mm when viewed from the proximal surface, or from labial to lingual. Both cusps are within the confines of the roots which helps to absorb some of the pressure from mastication.

The root trunk is bifurcated for one half its length. Both roots are straight until the apical third where they incline toward each other.

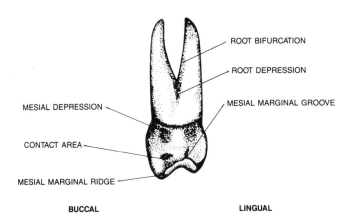

Figure 8-4 Maxillary first premolar—mesial surface

Mesial Surface. Extending from the occlusal surface and crossing the marginal ridge onto the mesial surface is a mesial marginal groove, Figure 8-4. At its end, only a short distance onto the mesial surface, is a mesial depression that continues onto the root and merges with the root bifurcation.

Distal Surface. The distal surface of the crown is smooth; it has no groove or depression. The root does have a depression that extends into the bifurcation, Figure 8-5.

Occlusal Surface. The occlusal shape forms a hexagon, circumscribed by the marginal and cusp ridges. Because the cusps tip inward, both the buccal and lingual surfaces are visible.

Note that the buccal cusp tip is centered between the mesial and distal sides, Figure 8-6. Both the buccal and lingual cusps are pyramid-shaped with their sides sloping toward the central groove and fossae. The slope from the tip of the buccal cusp to the central groove, and from the tip of the lingual cusp to the central groove, forms a triangular ridge. The two fossae are the mesial triangular and distal triangular fossa.

Located at the base of the cusps, and separating them, are the grooves. Although there can be several supplementary grooves, the major groove pattern common to all maxillary first premolars includes the central, mesio-buccal, disto-buccal, mesio-marginal, and disto-lingual grooves, Figure 8-6. As with most occlusal patterns, these structures are named by their location.

It is common to find a pit where two or more grooves merge. Thus, it is likely that this occlusal will have a mesial and distal pit located in the fossae.

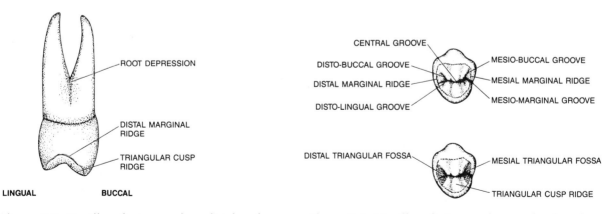

Figure 8-5 Maxillary first premolar—distal surface

Figure 8-6 Maxillary first premolar—occlusal surface

Summary of the Maxillary First Premolar

Buccal Surface. The characteristics of this surface are:

- A prominent buccal ridge.
- A pointed buccal cusp.
- A mesial side that is concave from the cervix to the contact area; a contact area that is in the middle of the surface; a cusp slope that is straighter and longer than the distal.
- A distal side that is straight from the cervix to the contact area; a contact area that is more occlusal than on the mesial; a cusp slope that is shorter than the mesial.
- The buccal root only is visible.

Lingual Surface. The characteristics of this surface are:

- Both cusps visible.
- A smooth lingual cusp that is shorter and narrower than the buccal cusp.
- Visible mesial and distal surfaces.

Proximal Surfaces. The characteristics of these surfaces are:

- Two visible cusps; a lingual cusp that is 1 mm shorter than the buccal cusp.
- Two visible roots. (Two pulp canals)
- Cusps that are within the confines of the root trunk.
- A mesial crown surface with a mesial marginal groove and a mesial developmental depression that extends from the crown to the root bifurcation.
- A distal surface with no grooves and no depressions.
- Both roots are straight until the apical third, then incline toward each other.
- Root bifurcates for one half its length.

Occlusal Surface. The characteristics of this surface are:

- Visible buccal and lingual surfaces.
- A buccal cusp centered between the mesial and distal side.

- Fossae: mesial and distal triangular.
- Grooves: central, mesio-buccal, mesio-marginal, disto-buccal, and disto-lingual.

MAXILLARY SECOND PREMOLAR

CHARACTERISTICS
  LOCATION IN THE ARCH . . . . Fifth tooth from the midline; distal to the first premolar
  UNIVERSAL NUMBER . . . . R-#4   L-#13
  ERUPTION DATE . . . . 10-12 years
  FIRST EVIDENCE OF CALCIFICATION . . . . 2 years
  CROWN COMPLETION . . . . 6-7 years
  ROOT COMPLETION . . . . 12-14 years
  FUNCTION . . . . Grinding
  LENGTH OF CROWN . . . . 8.5 mm
  LENGTH OF ROOT . . . . 14 mm
  ANTAGONISTS . . . . Mandibular second premolar and first molar

LOCATION OF CONTACT AREA
  MESIAL . . . . Middle of the tooth
  DISTAL . . . . Middle of the tooth

IDENTIFYING FEATURES
  - two cusps: one buccal, one lingual
  - one root, one pulp canal
  - resembles first premolar with slight variations

(Refer to Figure 8-7 on page 92.)

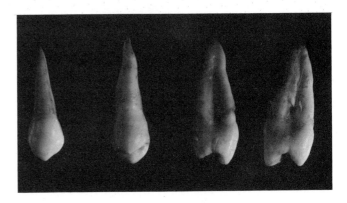

Figure 8-7 Maxillary second premolar

Tooth Description of the Maxillary Second Premolar

The maxillary second premolar (Figure 8-8) looks like the maxillary first premolar but has the following variations:

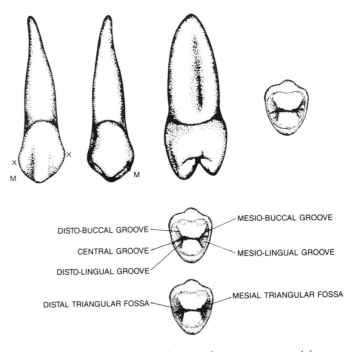

Figure 8-8 Maxillary second premolar—grooves and fossae

- There is only one root and one pulp canal.
- The mesial buccal cusp slope is shorter than the distal buccal cusp slope.
- Both cusps are about the same length (lingual slightly shorter).
- The mesial surface of the crown has no groove and no depression. From the occlusal view, there may be a mesial marginal groove but it seldom extends onto the mesial surface, Figure 8-9.
- A shallow depression is evident on the mesial root.

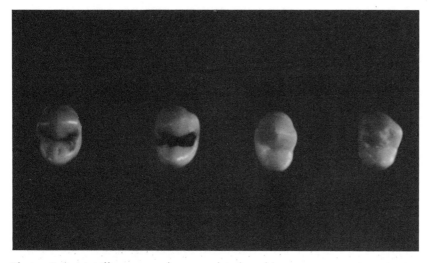

Figure 8-9 Maxillary premolars—occlusal surfaces

SUMMARY

Maxillary premolars are positioned just distal to the maxillary canines. There are two in each maxillary quadrant. Each premolar has two cusps, a buccal and a lingual, which accounts for their alternate designation of bicuspids. An occlusal surface lies between the cusps and this surface is used to crush and grind the food in its preparation for digestion.

Premolars replace deciduous molars. These teeth, along with the molars, are considered posterior teeth.

The maxillary first premolars have two roots; the second premolar has only one. Because of their similarities, the roots are usually the only way to distinguish the first from the second premolar.

WORKSHEET

A. Complete the chart with the information requested.

	MAXILLARY FIRST PREMOLAR	MAXILLARY SECOND PREMOLAR
Universal Number		
Palmer's Notation		
Eruption Date		
Antagonists		
Succedaneous		
Number of Cusps		
Number of Roots		
Identifying Features* Buccal		
Lingual		
Mesial		
Distal		
Occlusal Description Cusps		
Fossae		
Grooves		

*Size, no. of cusps; location of grooves, etc.

9

Mandibular Premolars

GENERAL INFORMATION
MANDIBULAR FIRST PREMOLAR
MANDIBULAR SECOND PREMOLAR

Objectives

- Identify the mandibular premolars and provide vital information: i.e., universal number, function, antagonist, etc.
- Describe the location and contour of each mandibular premolar.
- Define the new terms in the chapter.
- Complete the worksheet at the end of the chapter.

GENERAL INFORMATION

There are four mandibular premolars: two in each quadrant. They are named by their position in the arch from anterior to posterior as first premolar and second premolar.

The mandibular first premolar has one buccal and one lingual cusp. Differing from the others, the mandibular second premolar often has one buccal and two lingual cusps; it is the only premolar with three cusps.

Both mandibular premolars have one root. Mandibular premolars assist the maxillary premolars with grinding and chewing food.

MANDIBULAR FIRST PREMOLAR

CHARACTERISTICS

LOCATION IN THE ARCH . . . . Fourth tooth from the midline;
distal to canine

UNIVERSAL NUMBER . . . . R-#28   L-#21

ERUPTION DATE . . . . 10-12 years

FIRST EVIDENCE OF CALCIFICATION . . . . 1¼-2 years

CROWN COMPLETION . . . . 5-6 years

ROOT COMPLETION . . . . 12-13 years

FUNCTION . . . . Grinding

LENGTH OF CROWN . . . . 8.5 mm

LENGTH OF ROOT . . . . 14 mm

ANTAGONISTS . . . . Maxillary cuspid and first
premolar

LOCATION OF CONTACT AREA

MESIAL . . . . Middle of the tooth

DISTAL . . . . Middle of the tooth

IDENTIFYING FEATURES

- two cusps: one buccal, one lingual
- lingual cusp is small and nonfunctioning
- one root; sometimes it tends to bifurcate at the apex
- mesio-lingual groove

(Refer to Figure 9-1.)

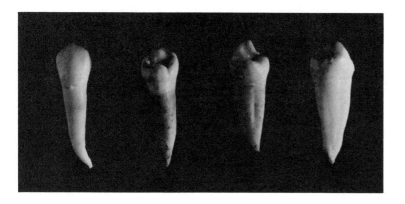

Figure 9-1 Mandibular first premolar

Tooth Description of the Mandibular First Premolar

Buccal Surface. A very prominent buccal ridge, perhaps more rounded than any of the other premolars, extends to a pointed cusp, Figure 9-2. Again, as was evident in the maxillary premolars, shallow depression occurs on either side of the buccal ridge. The mesial cusp slope is shorter than the distal.

The *mesial side* is concave from the cervix to the rounded contact area in the middle of the surface. The *distal* outline is also slightly concave from the cervix to the contact area, about in the middle of the tooth.

The cervix is narrow. The root is tapered and about 3-4 mm shorter than the adjacent cuspid.

Figure 9-2 Mandibular first premolar—buccal surface

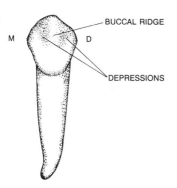

M   D

BUCCAL RIDGE

DEPRESSIONS

Lingual Surface. The lingual cusp is short and poorly developed, extending only two-thirds the height of the crown, Figure 9-3. It is a *nonfunctioning* cusp. Because of the position of the cusps, most of the occlusal surface can be seen from this view. Extending from the occlusal surface onto the lingual is a mesio-lingual groove which delineates the lingual cusp.

Mesial Surface. Both the buccal and lingual cusps, as well as some of the occlusal surface, are seen, Figure 9-4. The tip of the buccal cusp is centered over the root. Parallel to the buccal triangular ridge is the mesio-marginal ridge which is interrupted, or broken, by the mesio-lingual groove.

A broad root, tapering only at the apical third, has a deep developmental groove near the apex. Often this groove will bifurcate the tip of the root.

Distal Surface. The overall shape is the reverse of the mesial but the surface structures vary. The distal marginal ridge is perpendicular to the buccal cusp ridge and there is no interruption by grooves, Figure 9-5. The root has a shallow depression, but there is seldom a groove near the apical third.

Occlusal View. Most of the buccal surface can be seen from this view (Figure 9-6), as well as the following occlusal structures:

- Fossae (both irregular in shape): mesial, distal
- Grooves: mesio-buccal, disto-buccal, mesio-lingual

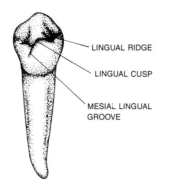

Figure 9-3 Mandibular first premolar—lingual surface

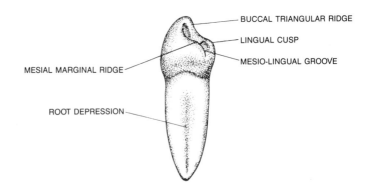

Figure 9-4 Mandibular first premolar—mesial surface

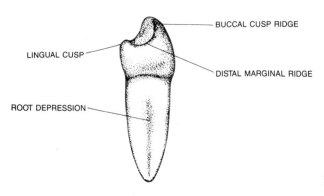
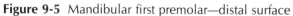

Figure 9-5 Mandibular first premolar—distal surface

A variation of the groove pattern may show a central groove between the mesio-buccal and the disto-buccal, Figure 9-7.

Summary of the Mandibular First Premolar

Buccal Surface. The characteristics of this surface are:

- A prominent buccal ridge.
- A pointed cusp.
- A narrow cervix.
- A mesial side that is concave from the cervix to the contact area; a contact area at the middle of the tooth; a mesial cusp slope shorter than the distal.
- A distal that is concave from the cervix to the contact area; a contact area that is in the middle of the tooth; a cusp slope that is longer than the mesial.

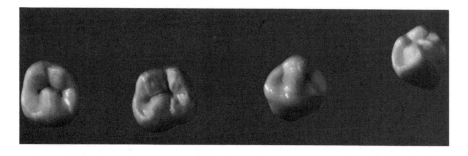

Figure 9-6 Mandibular premolars—occlusal surfaces

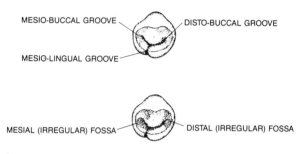

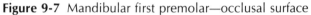

Figure 9-7 Mandibular first premolar—occlusal surface

Lingual Surface. The characteristics of this surface are:

- Visible mesial and distal surfaces.
- A short lingual cusp that is two-thirds the height of the crown.
- A lingual cusp that is nonfunctioning.
- A mesio-lingual groove that delineates the lingual cusp.

Proximal Surfaces. The characteristics of this surface are:

- Both cusps visible.
- The tip of the buccal cusp is centered over the root.
- A visible occlusal surface.
- A mesial surface with a mesio-marginal ridge that is parallel to the buccal triangular ridge; a mesio-lingual groove that interrupts the mesio-marginal ridge; a slight curve in the cervical line; a broad root with a deep developmental groove at the apical third.
- A distal surface with a distal marginal ridge that is perpendicular to the buccal cusp ridge; a marginal ridge that is uninterrupted; a root that has a shallow depression but seldom has a groove; a cervical line that is straight; a concavity on the surface near the cervical line.

Occlusal Surface. The characteristics of this surface are:

- A visible buccal surface.
- Two irregular fossae: mesial and distal.
- Grooves: mesio-buccal, disto-buccal, and mesio-lingual.

MANDIBULAR SECOND PREMOLAR

CHARACTERISTICS

LOCATION IN THE ARCH . . . . Fifth tooth from midline; distal to
first premolar

UNIVERSAL NUMBER . . . . R-#29   L-#20

ERUPTION DATE . . . . 11-12 years

FIRST EVIDENCE OF CALCIFICATION . . . . 2½ years

CROWN COMPLETION . . . . 6-7 years

ROOT COMPLETION . . . . 13-14 years

FUNCTION . . . . Grinding

LENGTH OF CROWN . . . . 8 mm

LENGTH OF ROOT . . . . 14.5 mm

ANTAGONISTS . . . . Maxillary first and second
premolar

LOCATION OF CONTACT AREA

MESIAL . . . . Middle of the tooth

DISTAL . . . . Middle of the tooth

IDENTIFYING FEATURES

- three cusps: buccal, mesio-lingual, disto-lingual

- one root, one pulp canal

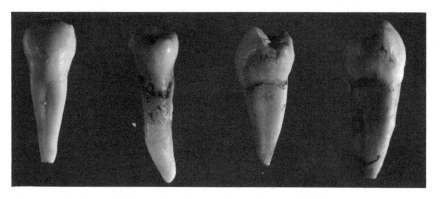

Figure 9-8 Mandibular second premolar

Tooth Description of the Mandibular Second Premolar

The following description is of a mandibular second premolar with three cusps: the buccal, mesio-lingual, and disto-lingual. When the mandibular second premolar has only two cusps, it resembles the mandibular first premolar.

Buccal Surface. From the buccal view the second premolar looks similar to the first premolar but it is slightly broader and shorter with contact areas a bit more occlusal than the first premolar. Only the buccal cusp is visible.

Lingual Surface. All three cusps are visible because the lingual cusps are shorter than the buccal cusp. Both lingual cusps are functioning cusps. Separating the two lingual cusps is the lingual groove, Figure 9-9. The mesio-lingual cusp is the larger of the two lingual cusps.

Mesial Surface. Since the mesial side of the tooth is larger than the distal, only the buccal and mesio-lingual cusps are visible, Figure 9-10. The mesial marginal ridge forms a right angle with the buccal cusp slope; it is not broken by a groove. The mesial surface is smooth, with only a slight curvature at the cervical line. The root is broad, tapering at the apical third.

Distal Surface. Because the teeth converge toward the posterior portion of the mouth, the distal of the tooth is narrower than the mesial, revealing some of the occlusal surface. All three cusps can be seen, Figure 9-11.

Occlusal Surface. In order of size, from largest to smallest, the cusps are buccal, mesio-lingual, and disto-lingual. The cusps are divided by grooves forming a "Y"

Figure 9-9 Mandibular second premolar—lingual surface

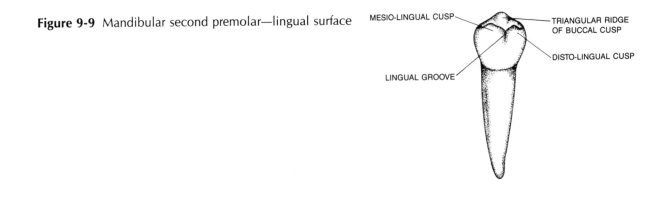

MESIO-LINGUAL CUSP

TRIANGULAR RIDGE OF BUCCAL CUSP

DISTO-LINGUAL CUSP

LINGUAL GROOVE

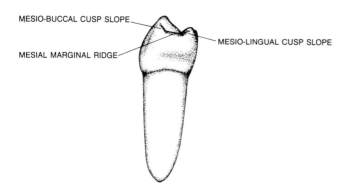

Figure 9-10 Mandibular second premolar—mesial surface

shaped pattern, Figure 9-12. There are two fossae, both triangular in shape: mesial and distal triangular fossae.

Summary of the Mandibular Second Premolar

Buccal Surface. The characteristics of this surface are:

- A resemblance to the first premolar but slightly shorter and broader.
- Contact areas that are in the middle of the tooth but slightly more occlusal than the first premolar.

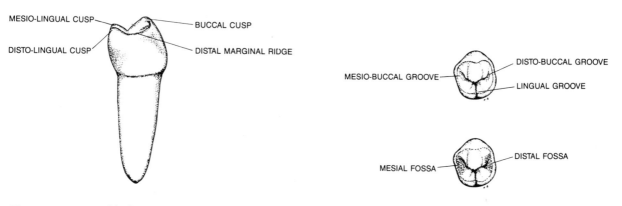

Figure 9-11 Mandibular second premolar—distal surface

Figure 9-12 Mandibular second premolar—occlusal surface

Lingual Surface. The characteristics of this surface are:

- Three visible cusps: buccal, mesio-lingual, and disto-lingual.
- Cusps that are all functioning.
- Lingual cusps that are shorter than the buccal cusp.
- A lingual groove that divides the two lingual cusps.

Proximal Surfaces. The characteristics of these surfaces are:

- A mesial surface with visible buccal and mesio-lingual cusps; a mesial marginal ridge that forms a right angle with the buccal cusp slope; a cervical line that has a slight curvature.
- A distal surface having more of the occlusal surface visible; all three cusps visible.
- The order of the cusp size is: buccal-1; mesio-lingual-2; disto-lingual-3.
- A broad root tapering at the apical third.

Occlusal Surface. The characteristics of this surface are:

- Two triangular fossae: mesial and distal.
- Mesio-buccal, disto-buccal, and lingual grooves.
- Grooves that form a "Y" shape.

SUMMARY

Mandibular premolars are positioned just distal to the mandibular canines. There are two in each mandibular quadrant. Although the first premolar has two cusps, the second premolar frequently has three cusps; consequently, the term *bicuspid* would not be appropriate for this tooth.

The mandibular first premolar has not only a sharp, pointed buccal cusp but also a short, non-functioning lingual cusp that makes this tooth easy to distinguish from other premolars. The mandibular second premolar may resemble the first, but it frequently has three cusps (one buccal and two lingual) that are nearly the same height.

As with all posterior teeth, the occlusal surface is located between the cusps and outlined by marginal ridges. All cusps slope into grooves located at the base of the occlusal surface.

WORKSHEET

A. Complete the chart with the information requested.

	FIRST PREMOLAR	SECOND PREMOLAR
Universal Number		
Palmer's Notation		
Eruption Date		
Antagonists		
Succedaneous		
Number of Cusps		
Number of Roots		
Identifying Features* Buccal		
Lingual		
Mesial		
Distal		
Occlusal Description Cusps		
Fossae		
Grooves		

*Size, no. of cusps; location of grooves, etc.

B. On the drawings below, draw and label the grooves and fossae for each premolar.

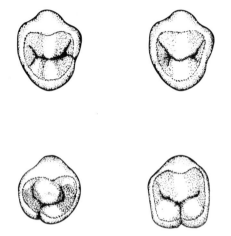

C. Put the letter of the correct answer in the space provided below.
The answer can include more than one letter.

    a. Max. first premolar   c. Mand. first premolar   e. none
    b. Max. second premolar   d. Mand. second premolar   f. all

_____First evidence of calcification occurs between 2-2½ years.

_____Eruption takes place between ages 10 and 11.

_____Occludes with the mandibular first and second premolar.

_____Mesial marginal ridge is interrupted.

_____Has a central groove.

_____Has a "Y" shaped occlusal groove pattern.

_____The distal marginal ridge is continuous.

_____Has a nonfunctioning cusp.

_____Has three cusps.

_____Is a succedaneous tooth.

_____Middle buccal lobe is well developed.

_____Has two pulp canals.

_____Lingual cusp can be seen from the buccal.

_____Has irregular fossa.

_____Develops from five lobes.

10

Maxillary First and Second Molars

Objectives

- Identify the maxillary first and second molars and provide vital information: i.e., universal number, function, antagonist, etc.
- Describe the location and contour of each first and second maxillary molar.
- Define new terms in the chapter.
- Complete the worksheet at the end of the chapter.

GENERAL INFORMATION

There are six maxillary molars: three in each quadrant. Like the premolars, molars are named by their position in the arch from anterior to posterior or first molar, second molar, and third molar. Permanent molars erupt posterior to the deciduous second molars and do not replace deciduous teeth.

The first molar is the first permanent tooth to erupt. The mandibular first molar precedes the maxillary first molar by a few months, but both usually erupt before the permanent central incisors.

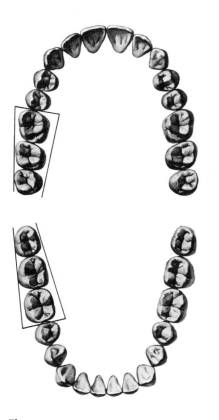

Figure 10-1 Posterior teeth converge toward the distal, or the mesial surface is wider than the distal (Base art copyright by the American Dental Association. Reprinted by permission.)

All maxillary molars have at least four cusps. The maxillary first molar usually has a fifth, nonfunctioning cusp, or tubercle, that is positioned on another cusp. The number of lobes from which a molar develops is the same as the number of cusps.

Maxillary molars have *trifurcated* (divided into three) roots: mesio-buccal, disto-buccal, and lingual. Each root has one pulp canal.

Molars are structured so that they are narrower, or converge, toward the posterior portion of the mouth. Thus, the distal of the tooth is narrower than the mesial as shown in Figure 10-1. Because they have multi-cusps, molars perform the major task of mastication by grinding and pulverizing food.

MAXILLARY FIRST MOLAR

CHARACTERISTICS
  LOCATION IN THE ARCH . . . . Sixth tooth from midline; distal to
                                                                      maxillary second premolar
  UNIVERSAL NUMBER . . . . R-#3   L-#14
  ERUPTION DATE . . . . 6-7 years
  FIRST EVIDENCE OF CALCIFICATION . . . . Birth
  CROWN COMPLETION . . . . 2½-3 years
  ROOT COMPLETION . . . . 9-10 years
  FUNCTION . . . . Mastication and comminution of
                                                                      food
  LENGTH OF CROWN . . . . 7.5 mm
  LENGTH OF ROOT . . . . 12 mm buccal
                                                                      13 mm lingual
  ANTAGONISTS . . . . Mandibular first and second molars

LOCATION OF CONTACT AREA
  MESIAL . . . . 2/3 distance from cervical line
  DISTAL . . . . Middle of the tooth

IDENTIFYING FEATURES
  • five cusps: mesio-buccal, disto-buccal, mesio-lingual, disto-lingual, cusp of Carabelli
  • three roots: mesio-buccal, disto-buccal, lingual
  • three pulp canals, one in each root
  • cusp of Carabelli, or fifth cusp, located on the mesio-lingual cusp, is a nonfunctioning cusp
  • largest and strongest of the maxillary teeth

(Refer to Figure 10-2.)

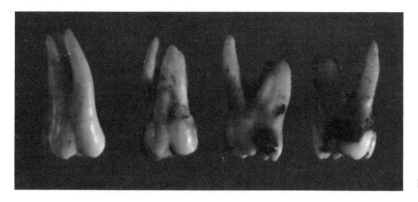

Figure 10-2 Maxillary first molar

Tooth Description of the Maxillary First Molar

Buccal Surface. The two buccal cusps and the cusp tips of the two longer lingual cusps are seen from this view, Figure 10-3. Dividing the mesio-buccal and disto-buccal cusps is the buccal groove. This extends about one half the length of the crown, ending in a shallow depression.

The mesial side, from cervix to contact area, is straight. The contact area, located about two-thirds the distance from the cervical line, is convex. The distal side is convex and reaches the contact area in the middle of the tooth. The cervical line forms a slight curve.

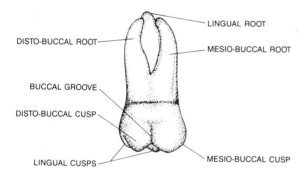

Figure 10-3 Maxillary right first molar—buccal view

Before bifurcating into a mesio-buccal and disto-buccal root, the root trunk extends about 4 mm. A shallow depression continues from the cervical line to its end as a deep groove at the bifurcation. The mesio-buccal root extends halfway in a mesial direction before curving distally; the smaller disto-buccal root is straight for half its length, then curves mesially. Seen between the two buccal roots and extending above them by 1 mm is the lingual root.

Lingual Surface. Since the two lingual cusps, mesio-lingual and disto-lingual, are longer than the buccal cusps, they block the buccal cusps from view. Dividing the two lingual cusps is the lingual groove, Figure 10-4. The mesio-lingual cusp is about three-fifths the width of the crown and supports the fifth cusp, the cusp (or tubercle) of Carabelli. The mesio-lingual cusp is the largest cusp. The fifth cusp is not always present and when it is, it may not be well-developed since it is a nonfunctioning cusp. A short groove, the fifth cusp groove, is usually present on the mesio-lingual cusp when the tubercle is absent. The disto-lingual cusp is a smooth spheroid.

Although the lateral borders of the two buccal roots can be seen, the lingual root is dominant. It is broad with a furrow extending most of its length, and tapers to a blunt apex.

Mesial Surface. Because the mesial side is wider than the distal, only the mesio-buccal and mesio-lingual cusps and the cusp of Carabelli are seen, Figure 10-5. The mesio-marginal ridge, connecting the cusps, is about one fifth the distance from the cusp tips; it obstructs the occlusal surface. Just cervical to the contact area is a shallow depression that continues from the crown onto the root trunk.

Both the mesio-buccal and lingual root block the smaller distal root. The mesio-buccal root is flat, but broad, with a depression spanning most of its length. The lingual root is long and narrow, banana shaped, from this aspect, Figure 10-6.

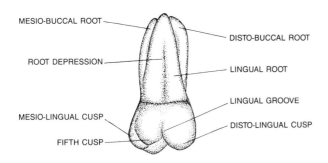

MESIO-BUCCAL ROOT

DISTO-BUCCAL ROOT

ROOT DEPRESSION

LINGUAL ROOT

LINGUAL GROOVE

MESIO-LINGUAL CUSP

DISTO-LINGUAL CUSP

FIFTH CUSP

Figure 10-4 Maxillary first molar—lingual surface

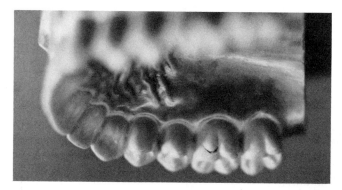

Figure 10-5 The cusp of Carabelli. (Courtesy of Nancy Somers)

Distal Surface. Because the crown converges, some of the buccal surface can be seen, Figure 10-7. The disto-marginal ridge curves more cervically than the mesial marginal ridge, exposing some of the occlusal surface.

The cervical line is almost straight. Although all three roots are visible, only the outline of the mesio-buccal root can be seen. From the cervical line to the disto-buccal root is a depression. There is no concavity at the bifurcation.

Occlusal Surface. The width from buccal to lingual is wider than from mesial to distal. Looking down onto the occlusal surface, it is easier to see the convergence of the crown toward the distal and the size of the five cusps. From largest to smallest, the cusps are mesio-lingual, mesio-buccal, disto-buccal, disto-lingual, and cusp of Carabelli.

The buccal groove extends from the buccal surface onto the occlusal and joins the central groove, Figure 10-8. The disto-buccal cusp and the mesio-lingual cusp, which form an oblique ridge, are divided by a transverse groove, an extension of the central groove which continues into the distal fossa. On the occlusal surface, the two lingual cusps are divided by the distal oblique groove which, obviously, extends obliquely into the distal fossa.

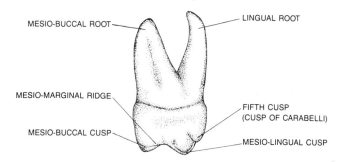

MESIO-BUCCAL ROOT

LINGUAL ROOT

MESIO-MARGINAL RIDGE

FIFTH CUSP (CUSP OF CARABELLI)

MESIO-BUCCAL CUSP

MESIO-LINGUAL CUSP

Figure 10-6 Maxillary first molar—mesial surface

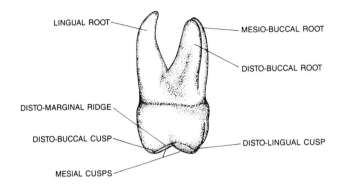

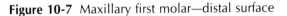

Figure 10-7 Maxillary first molar—distal surface

All cusps slope downward toward the grooves. It is the base of the slopes that form the fossa. On this tooth there is a large circular central fossa. Notice, on Figure 10-7, the number of cusps that slope into it. The two lingual cusps slope into the distal linear fossa as well as into the mesial or distal triangular fossa.

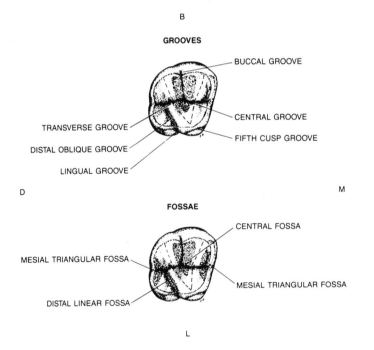

Figure 10-8 Maxillary first molar—occlusal surface

Summary of the Maxillary First Molar

Buccal Surface. The characteristics of this surface are:

Crown

- Two buccal cusps: mesio-buccal and disto-buccal.
- Two longer lingual cusp tips are visible.
- The buccal groove divides the two buccal cusps; it extends one-half the crown length and terminates in a shallow depression.
- The mesial outline is straight.
- The mesial contact is two-thirds the distance from the cervical line.
- The distal side is convex.
- The distal contact area is in the middle of the surface.

Root

- There are two buccal roots.
- The mesio-buccal root extends in a mesial direction for half its length and then curves distally.
- The disto-buccal root is straight for half its length, then curves mesially.
- The root trunk is about 4 mm long before bifurcating.
- A shallow depression extends from the cervical line and terminates in a deep groove at the bifurcation.
- The lingual root extends between and above the buccal roots.

Lingual Surface. The characteristics of this surface are:

Crown

- Three visible cusps: mesio-lingual, disto-lingual, cusp of Carabelli.
- A mesio-lingual cusp about three-fifths the width of the crown.
- A cusp of Carabelli positioned on the mesio-lingual cusp.
- A fifth cusp groove on the mesio-lingual cusp if the fifth cusp is not present.
- A lingual groove dividing the two lingual cusps.

Roots

- A broad, tapered lingual root, the longest of the three roots, with a furrow or depression.

- A visible outline of both buccal roots.

Mesial Surface. The characteristics of this surface are:

Crown

- Visible cusps: mesio-buccal, mesio-lingual, and cusp of Carabelli.
- A depression on the crown from the contact area to the root trunk.
- A mesio-marginal ridge about one-fifth the distance from the cusp tips.

Root

- Two visible roots: a broad, flat mesio-buccal root and a tapered lingual root.
- A depression on the lingual root.

Distal Surface. The characteristics of this surface are:

Crown

- Visible buccal and occlusal surfaces.
- An almost straight cervical line.

Root

- All three roots visible (only the border of the mesio-buccal root can be seen).
- A depression from the cervical line to the disto-buccal root.
- No concavity in the area; no root bifurcation.

Occlusal Surface. The characteristics of this surface are:

- Dimensions that are wider from the buccal to the lingual than from the mesial to the distal.
- Four functioning *cusps* and a small fifth cusp (in order of size): mesio-lingual, mesio-buccal, disto-buccal, disto-lingual, and cusp of Carabelli.
- Grooves: buccal, central, transverse groove of the oblique ridge, distal oblique; the lingual and fifth cusp groove are visible from this view.
- Fossae: central, distal linear, mesial triangular, and distal triangular.

MAXILLARY SECOND MOLAR

CHARACTERISTICS

LOCATION IN THE ARCH . . . . Seventh tooth from the midline; distal to first molar

UNIVERSAL NUMBER . . . . R-#2   L-#15

ERUPTION DATE . . . . 12-13 years

FIRST EVIDENCE OF CALCIFICATION . . . . 2½-3 years

CROWN COMPLETION . . . . 7-8 years

ROOT COMPLETION . . . . 14-16 years

FUNCTION . . . . Mastication and comminution

LENGTH OF CROWN . . . . 7 mm

LENGTH OF ROOT . . . . 11 mm buccal
12 mm lingual

ANTAGONISTS . . . . Mandibular second and third molars

LOCATION OF CONTACT AREA

MESIAL . . . . 2/3 from cervical line

DISTAL . . . . Middle of the tooth

IDENTIFYING FEATURES

- four cusps: mesio-buccal, disto-buccal, mesio-lingual, disto-lingual

- three roots: mesio-buccal, disto-buccal, lingual

- three pulp canals — one in each root

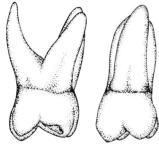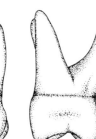

Figure 10-9 Maxillary second molar

Tooth Description of the Maxillary Second Molar

The maxillary second molar is similar to the maxillary first molar in size, shape, and function but has the following differences:

- Both crown and root are slightly smaller.
- The second molar has only four cusps: mesio-buccal, disto-buccal, mesio-lingual, and disto-lingual.
- There is no cusp of Carabelli.
- The roots are not as divergent.
- The occlusal surface has more supplementary grooves.
- There is no transverse groove of the oblique ridge.

Occlusal Surface. The characteristics of this surface, shown in Figure 10-10, are:

Grooves: buccal, lingual, and central

Fossae: central, distal linear, distal triangular, and mesial triangular

Cusps, in order of size: mesio-lingual, mesio-buccal, disto-buccal, and disto-lingual

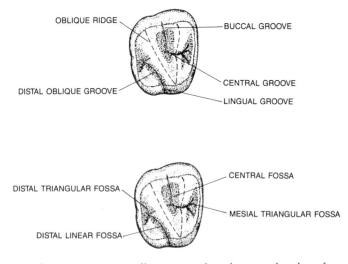

Figure 10-10 Maxillary second molar—occlusal surface

SUMMARY

There are three maxillary molars in each maxillary quadrant. They have at least four cusps and a broad occlusal surface. Because of their size, the molars perform the major task of grinding and pulverizing food.

The maxillary first molar has four functioning cusps and one small tubercle on the mesio-lingual cusp called the fifth cusp, or Cusp of Carabelli. The first molar is the largest and strongest of the maxillary teeth. The second molar resembles the first but does not have the fifth cusp, and its overall dimensions are slightly smaller than the first.

All maxillary molars have three roots, each with one pulp canal. Molars are not succedaneous teeth.

WORKSHEET

A. Complete the chart with the information requested.

	FIRST MOLAR	SECOND MOLAR
Universal Number		
Palmer's Notation		
Eruption Date		
Antagonists		
Succedaneous		
Number of Cusps		
Number of Roots		
Identifying Features* Buccal		

(Chart is continued on the following page.)

	FIRST MOLAR	SECOND MOLAR
Lingual		
Mesial		
Distal		
Occlusal Description Cusps		
Fossae		
Grooves		

*Size, no. of cusps; location of grooves, etc.

B. *Using the drawing below, draw and label the groove pattern and the fossae.*

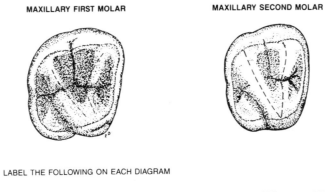

MAXILLARY FIRST MOLAR   MAXILLARY SECOND MOLAR

LABEL THE FOLLOWING ON EACH DIAGRAM

	GROOVES	FOSSAE	RIDGES	PIT
FIRST	BUCCAL CENTRAL TRANSVERSE DISTAL OBLIQUE LINGUAL	CENTRAL DISTAL TRIANGULAR MESIAL TRIANGULAR DISTAL LINEAR	MARGINAL OBLIQUE	
SECOND	ALL OF THE ABOVE *EXCEPT* THE TRANSVERSE	SAME AS ABOVE		

11

Mandibular First and Second Molars

GENERAL INFORMATION
MANDIBULAR FIRST MOLAR
MANDIBULAR SECOND MOLAR

Objectives

- Identify the mandibular first and second molars and provide vital information: i.e., universal number, function, antagonist, etc.
- Describe the location and contour of each first and second molar.
- Define new terms in the chapter.
- Complete the worksheet at the end of the chapter.

GENERAL INFORMATION

There are six mandibular molars: three in each quadrant. As with the maxillary molars, they are named for their position in the arch: first, second, and third molar. Again, molars erupt posterior to the deciduous second molars and are not succedaneous teeth.

The mandibular first molar is the first permanent tooth to erupt and its positioning in the arch is important for the appropriate alignment of the other permanent teeth. (See Chapter 15 - Occlusion) Therefore, it is considered the "keystone" of the dental arch.

Mandibular molars have either four or five cusps; the number of lobes from which they develop is the same as the number of cusps. The roots of mandibular molars are *bifurcated* (divided in two) into a mesial and distal root. Although each root of a tooth usually has one pulp canal, the mandibular first molar is the exception and has two pulp canals in the mesial root. The major function of the mandibular molars is to assist the maxillary molars with grinding and pulverizing the food.

MANDIBULAR FIRST MOLAR

CHARACTERISTICS
  LOCATION IN THE ARCH . . . . Sixth tooth from the midline; distal to second premolar
  UNIVERSAL NUMBER . . . . R-#30   L-#19
  ERUPTION DATE . . . . 6-7 years
  FIRST EVIDENCE OF CALCIFICATION . . . . Birth
  CROWN COMPLETION . . . . 2½-3 years
  ROOT COMPLETION . . . . 9-10 years
  FUNCTION . . . . Mastication and comminution of food
  LENGTH OF CROWN . . . . 7.5 mm
  LENGTH OF ROOT . . . . 14 mm
  ANTAGONISTS . . . . Maxillary second premolar and first molar

LOCATION OF CONTACT AREA
  MESIAL . . . . Occlusal third
  DISTAL . . . . Occlusal third

IDENTIFYING FEATURES
  • five cusps: mesio-buccal, disto-buccal, distal, mesio-lingual, disto-lingual
  • two roots: mesial and distal
  • three pulp canals: two in mesial root; one in distal root
  • largest mandibular tooth
  • first permanent tooth to erupt

(Refer to Figure 11-1.)

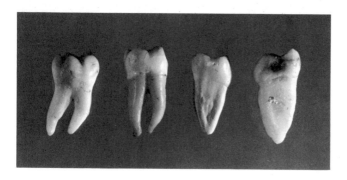

Figure 11-1 Mandibular first molar

Tooth Description of the Mandibular First Molar

Buccal Surface. Three buccal cusps and the tips of the two higher lingual cusps can be seen. The buccal cusps are flat and separated by grooves, Figure 11-2. The cusps, in order of size, are mesio-buccal, disto-buccal, and distal. They are divided by the mesio-buccal and disto-buccal groove, respectively. Slight depressions are at the base of each groove.

The *mesial side*, from cervix to contact area, is concave becoming convex at the contact area in the occlusal third. The *distal side* is straight from cervix to contact area where it becomes convex. The contact area is located slightly more toward the occlusal than on the mesial side.

The cervical line curves slightly in an apical direction. The root trunk, about 3 mm in length, bifurcates into a mesial and distal root. For half its length, the mesial root curves mesially, then it curves toward the distal. The distal root is less curved and slants in a distal direction.

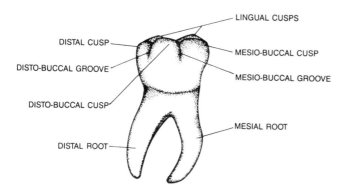

Figure 11-2 Mandibular right first molar—buccal surface

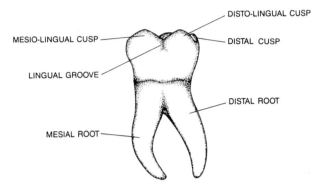

Figure 11-3 Mandibular first molar—lingual surface

Lingual Surface. There are two pointed lingual cusps, the mesio-lingual and disto-lingual, divided by a lingual groove, Figure 11-3. The distal cusp can also be seen. At the root bifurcation is a deep developmental groove.

Mesial Surface. Since the tooth is broader on the mesial side, only the mesio-buccal and mesio-lingual cusps are seen, Figure 11-4. They are joined by the mesial marginal ridge located about 1 mm below the cusp tips. The cervical line curves 1 mm in an occlusal direction.

Extending from the contact area and continuing onto the root is a shallow depression. The root remains broad for almost its entire length, tapering only at the apical third. This mesial root has *two pulp canals.*

Distal Surface. Because the crown converges toward the distal, a portion of the buccal surface is seen. The distal portion of the crown is also shorter so that all the cusps are visible, Figure 11-5. A relatively straight cervical line separates the crown and the root. A shallow depression is present on the distal root.

Figure 11-4 Mandibular first molar—mesial surface

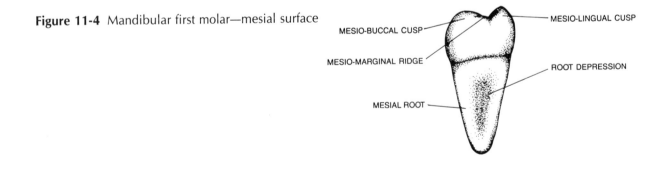

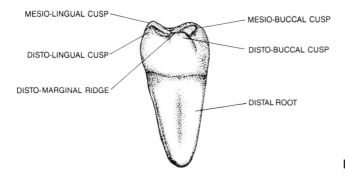

Figure 11-5 Mandibular first molar—distal surface

Occlusal Surface. The dimensions are wider from mesial to distal than from buccal to lingual, the opposite of the maxillary molar. All five cusps are functioning cusps, each separated by a groove, Figure 11-6. The occlusal grooves extend from the buccal and lingual surface and have the same names: mesio-buccal, disto-buccal, and lingual. They each join the central groove which goes from mesial to distal across the center of the occlusal surface. There is a deep central pit where grooves merge.

The sides of each cusp slope to form fossae. There is a large central circular fossa and mesial and distal triangular fossae.

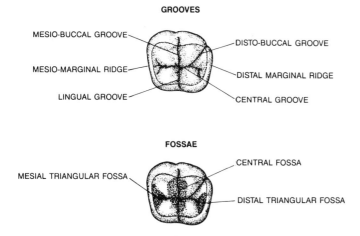

Figure 11-6 Mandibular right first molar—occlusal surface

Summary of the Mandibular First Molar

Buccal Surface. The characteristics of this surface are:

Crown

- Three flat buccal cusps: mesio-buccal, disto-buccal, and distal.
- Five cusps are visible since the lingual cusps are longer.
- Mesio-buccal and disto-buccal grooves divide the cusps.
- Slight depression at the base of the groove.
- A concave mesial side.
- A mesial contact area that is in the occlusal third.
- A straight distal side.
- A distal contact area that is more occlusal than mesial.

Root

- A mesial root that curves mesially; at midway, it curves distally.
- A distal root that is less curved, with its axis in a distal direction.
- A root that bifurcates about 3 mm below the cervical line and has a deep developmental depression.

Lingual Surface. The characteristics of this surface are:

Crown

- Two pointed lingual cusps: mesio-lingual and disto-lingual.
- A visible distal cusp.
- A lingual groove that divides the lingual cusps.

Roots

- A deep developmental depression at the root bifurcation.

Mesial Surface. The characteristics of this surface are:

Crown

- Two visible cusps: mesio-buccal and mesio-lingual.
- Mesio-marginal ridge located about 1 mm below cusp tips.
- Cervical line curves occlusally about 1 mm.
- Concave area at the cervical line that continues onto the root.

Root

- Only the mesial root is visible.
- Mesial root has two pulp canals.
- Broad and straight root, tapering in the apical third.
- A broad concavity or depression on the root.

Distal Surface. The characteristics of this surface are:

Crown

- Tooth converges toward distal so that some of the buccal surface is seen.
- Crown is shorter on the distal so that all cusps are seen.
- Relatively straight cervical line.

Root

- A shallow depression is often evident on the root.

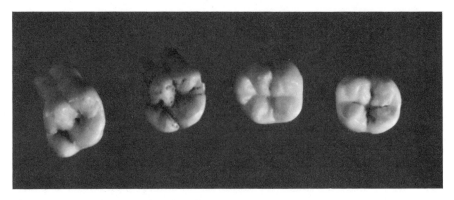

Figure 11-7 Molars—occlusal surfaces

Occlusal Surface. The characteristics of this surface are:

- Dimensions are wider (by 1 mm) from distal to mesial than from buccal to lingual, Figure 11-7.
- Five functioning cusps, in order of size, are mesio-lingual, mesio-buccal, disto-lingual, disto-buccal, and distal.
- Major grooves: central, mesio-buccal, disto-buccal, and lingual.
- Major fossae: central (circular), mesial, and distal triangular, Figure 11-8.
- Pits: central, mesial, and distal.

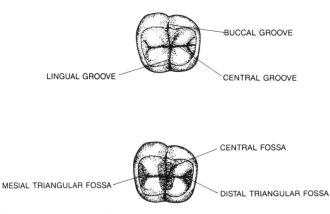

Figure 11-8 Mandibular second molar—occlusal surface

MANDIBULAR SECOND MOLAR

CHARACTERISTICS
    LOCATION IN THE ARCH . . . . Seventh tooth from the midline;
                                                                          distal to first molar
    UNIVERSAL NUMBER . . . . R-#31   L-#18
    ERUPTION DATE . . . . 11-13 years
    FIRST EVIDENCE OF CALCIFICATION . . . . 2½-3 years
    CROWN COMPLETION . . . . 7-8 years
    ROOT COMPLETION . . . . 14-15 years
    FUNCTION . . . . Mastication and comminution
    LENGTH OF CROWN . . . . 7 mm
    LENGTH OF ROOT . . . . 13 mm
    ANTAGONISTS . . . . Maxillary first and second molars

LOCATION OF CONTACT AREA
    MESIAL . . . . Occlusal third
    DISTAL . . . . Occlusal third
IDENTIFYING FEATURES
    • four cusps: mesio-buccal, disto-buccal, mesio-lingual, disto-lingual

    • two roots: mesial and distal

    • two pulp canals: one in each root

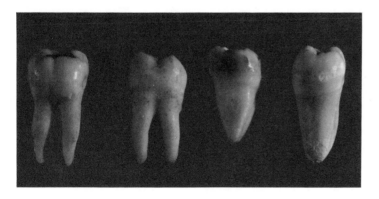

Figure 11-9 Mandibular second molar

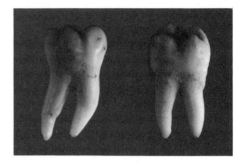

Figure 11-10 Mandibular first and second molars

Tooth Description of the Mandibular Second Molar

Because of its similarity to the first molar, only the structural variations are listed below, Figure 11-10.

- It is smaller.
- There are only four cusps: mesio-buccal, disto-buccal, mesio-lingual, disto-lingual.
- The buccal groove divides the two buccal cusps and continues onto the occlusal surface.
- The lingual groove divides the two lingual cusps and continues onto the occlusal surface.
- The mesial side of the tooth is wider (from buccal to lingual) than the distal. Therefore the mesial cusps are larger than the distal cusps.
- The occlusal groove pattern, shown in Figure 11-9, forms ⊣ ← buccal / ← central / ← lingual
- The occlusal has more supplementary grooves.
- The mesial root has only one pulp canal.

SUMMARY

Each mandibular quadrant has three mandibular molars. The mandibular first molar is usually the first permanent tooth to erupt, so it's positioning is important for the appropriate alignment of the other permanent teeth. Thus, it is the "keystone" to the arch.

The mandibular first molar has five cusps, three buccal and two lingual; the second molar has four cusps, two buccal and two lingual.

Mandibular molars have two roots, one mesial and one distal. All teeth have one pulp canal in each root, but the mandibular first molar is the exception. There are three pulp canals in the two roots: the mesial root has two pulp canals, the distal root has one pulp canal. The mandibular second molar has only one pulp canal in each root.

The mandibular molars assist the maxillary molars in mastication.

WORKSHEET

A. Complete the chart with the information requested.

	FIRST MOLAR	SECOND MOLAR
Universal Number		
Palmer's Notation		
Eruption Date		
Antagonists		
Succedaneous		
Number of Cusps		
Number of Roots		
Identifying Features* Buccal		
Lingual		
Mesial		
Distal		
Occlusal Description Cusps		
Fossae		
Grooves		

*Size, no. of cusps, location of grooves, etc.

B. Complete the figures, as described.

1. On the drawings below draw in the pulp canal(s).

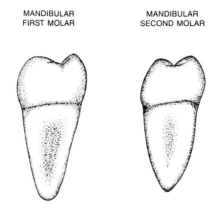

MANDIBULAR
FIRST MOLAR

MANDIBULAR
SECOND MOLAR

2. Using the drawing below draw and label the groove pattern and the fossae.

FIRST MOLAR

SECOND MOLAR

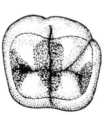

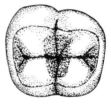

	GROOVES	**FOSSAE**	**RIDGES**	**PIT**
First	Central Mesio-buccal Disto-buccal Lingual	Central Mesial triangular Distal triangular	Marginal cusp	Central
Second	Central Buccal Lingual	same as above	same as above	

C. *Answer the following questions using the groove patterns for all molars that are shown below.*

MAXILLARY FIRST MOLAR

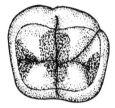

MAXILLARY SECOND MOLAR

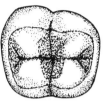

MAJOR:

GROOVES	FOSSAE	RIDGES
CENTRAL	CENTRAL	MARGINAL
DISTO-BUCCAL (FIRST ONLY)	MESIAL TRIANGULAR	CUSP
MESIO-BUCCAL (FIRST ONLY)	DISTAL TRIANGULAR	**PITS**
LINGUAL		CENTRAL PIT (FIRST ONLY)
BUCCAL (SECOND ONLY)		

MANDIBULAR FIRST MOLAR

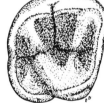

MANDIBULAR SECOND MOLAR

MAJOR:

GROOVES	FOSSAE	RIDGES
BUCCAL	CENTRAL	MARGINAL
BUCCAL GROOVE OF CENTRAL FOSSA	MESIAL TRIANGULAR	CUSP
CENTRAL	DISTAL TRIANGULAR	OBLIQUE
TRANSVERSE GROOVE OF THE OBLIQUE RIDGE	DISTAL LINEAR	MARGINAL
DISTAL OBLIQUE (FIRST ONLY)		
LINGUAL		
FIFTH CUSP GROOVE (FIRST ONLY)		

1. From the facial aspect of the mandibular molar, how many cusps are visible?

2. At age 11, what is the seventh tooth from the midline in the maxillary arch?

3. On which cusp of which tooth is the cusp of Carabelli located?

4. The largest cusp of the maxillary first molar is_____.

5. The oblique ridge of the maxillary first molar, occlusal surface extends between which cusps?

6. Name the roots of the maxillary molars.

7. Which occlusal groove is present on the maxillary first molar that is not on the maxillary second molar?

8. Name the fossae of the mandibular molars.

9. Which groove is found on the mandibular first molar that is not present on the mandibular second molar?

10. Which permanent tooth is the keystone to the arch, and why?

12

Third Molars

GENERAL INFORMATION
MAXILLARY THIRD MOLAR
MANDIBULAR THIRD MOLAR

Objectives

- Identify the third molars and provide vital information: i.e., universal number, function, antagonist, etc.
- Describe the location and contour of each third molar.
- Define new terms in the chapter.
- Complete the worksheet at the end of the chapter.

GENERAL INFORMATION

Because both maxillary and mandibular third molars show considerable developmental variation, there is no standard structural description. These teeth, more than any of the others, are likely to be anomalies. Often, there is crown displacement and the roots are fused or malformed.

When the third molars develop properly, their structure will look like either the first or second molar, but they can be differentiated because they are smaller and will have numerous supplementary grooves on the occlusal surface. The root will usually be fused even when the crown is not malformed.

Third molars supplement the other molars in grinding food. Although it is not necessary to study the structure of third molars, it is helpful to examine specimens to realize their difference from other molars.

MAXILLARY THIRD MOLAR

CHARACTERISTICS
    LOCATION IN THE ARCH . . . . Eighth tooth from midline; distal to
                                                                       maxillary second molar
    UNIVERSAL NUMBER . . . . R-#1   L-#16
    ERUPTION DATE . . . . .17-21 years
    FIRST EVIDENCE OF CALCIFICATION . . . . .7-9 years
    CROWN COMPLETION . . . . .12-16 years
    ROOT COMPLETION . . . . .18-25 years
    FUNCTION . . . . .Mastication and comminution
    LENGTH OF CROWN . . . . .6.5 mm
    LENGTH OF ROOT . . . . .11 mm
    ANTAGONISTS . . . . .Mandibular third molar

LOCATION OF CONTACT AREA
    MESIAL . . . . .variation from middle to
    DISTAL . . . . .occlusal third

IDENTIFYING FEATURES
    • often the crown is heart-shaped
    • fused roots (three roots)
    • may resemble first or second molar

MANDIBULAR THIRD MOLAR

CHARACTERISTICS
    LOCATION IN THE ARCH . . . . Eighth tooth from midline; distal to
                                                                       mandibular second molar
    UNIVERSAL NUMBER . . . . R-#32   L-#17
    ERUPTION DATE . . . . .17-21 years
    FIRST EVIDENCE OF CALCIFICATION . . . . .8-10 years

(Chart continued on following page)

CROWN COMPLETION . . . . .12-16 years
ROOT COMPLETION . . . . .18-25 years
FUNCTION . . . . .Mastication and comminution
LENGTH OF CROWN . . . . .7 mm
LENGTH OF ROOT . . . . .11 mm
ANTAGONISTS . . . . .Maxillary second and third molars

LOCATION OF CONTACT AREA
MESIAL . . . . .variation from middle to
DISTAL . . . . .occlusal third

IDENTIFYING FEATURES
- often crowns do not conform to normal size
- often have fused roots
- when well developed it will look like first or second molar

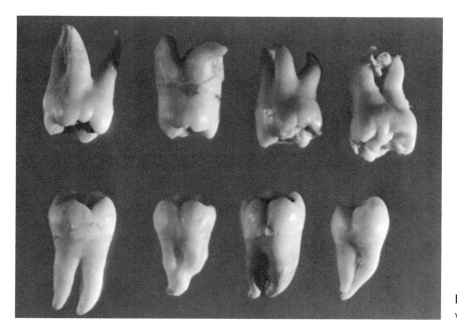

Figure 12-1 Developmental variations of third molars

SUMMARY

Because of developmental variations, there is no standard description for the maxillary or mandibular third molars. When they are well-formed, they will be smaller than but similar to the first molars in number of cusps and roots. Usually, however, the roots are fused and the crowns will have numerous supplementary grooves. Frequently, the maxillary third molar is heart-shaped, but the mandibular third molar is often atypical.

WORKSHEET

Answer the following questions as completely as possible:

1. What is the most common shape of the crown of the maxillary third molar?

2. What is a common feature of the roots of both maxillary and mandibular third molars?

3. When maxillary and mandibular molars develop normally, what do they resemble?

SECTION FOUR
RELATED TOPICS

13

Deciduous Dentition

THE NAMES AND NUMBER OF THE DECIDUOUS TEETH
ERUPTION/EXFOLIATION
COMPARISON WITH PERMANENT TEETH
DESCRIPTION OF DECIDUOUS TEETH
IMPORTANCE OF DECIDUOUS TEETH

Objectives

- Identify the names, number, and eruption dates of the deciduous teeth.
- Describe the value of the deciduous teeth to function.
- Compare the deciduous teeth to the permanent teeth.
- Complete the worksheet at the end of the chapter.

THE NAMES AND NUMBER OF THE DECIDUOUS TEETH

There are twenty deciduous teeth: ten maxillary and ten mandibular. In each quadrant there is a central incisor, lateral incisor, canine, first molar, and second molar, Figure 13-1. There are no premolars in the deciduous dentition. Deciduous teeth are also referred to as primary teeth, baby teeth, milk teeth, or first teeth.

ERUPTION/EXFOLIATION

The period of eruption for the deciduous teeth occurs from 6 months to 2½-3 years of age. The specific eruption date for each tooth is listed in Appendix A. All the deciduous teeth usually have emerged and are in alignment by the time

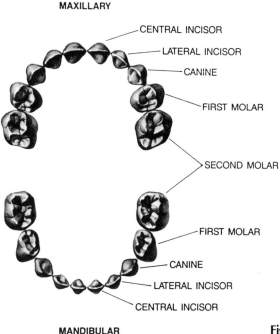

MAXILLARY

CENTRAL INCISOR

LATERAL INCISOR

CANINE

FIRST MOLAR

SECOND MOLAR

FIRST MOLAR

CANINE

LATERAL INCISOR

CENTRAL INCISOR

MANDIBULAR

Figure 13-1 Deciduous dentition (Base art copyright by the American Dental Association. Reprinted by permission.)

the child is 3 years old. Although each permanent tooth contacts its proximal tooth, there is spacing between each anterior deciduous tooth. This spacing allows for the development and growth of the larger succedaneous tooth forming in the bone beneath each deciduous tooth.

At 6 years, just prior to the eruption of the permanent mandibular central incisor, exfoliation of the deciduous teeth begins. The mandibular central incisors are the first to exfoliate. The exfoliation sequence is the same as the eruption sequence of the permanent dentition.

During the period when both deciduous and permanent teeth are present in the oral cavity, the person has a *mixed dentition*. By about 12 years of age, all deciduous teeth will be replaced by permanent teeth.

COMPARISON WITH PERMANENT TEETH

All deciduous teeth look like their permanent counterpart, although they are smaller, Figure 13-2. In contrast to the permanent teeth, the deciduous teeth appear whiter. Unless there is a mixed dentition, this is not as noticeable.

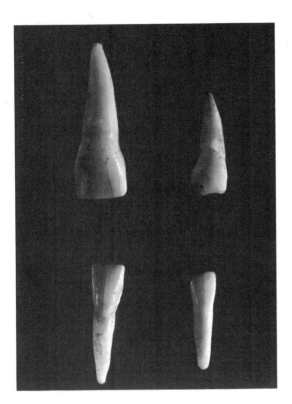

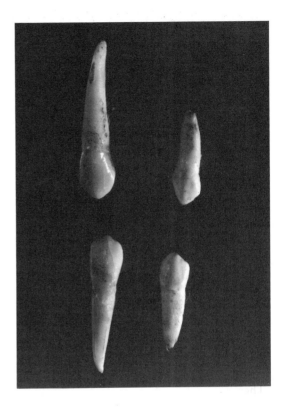

Figure 13-2 Deciduous incisors compared to permanent incisors

Figure 13-3 Deciduous canines compared to permanent canines

The deciduous teeth have a more pronounced cervical ridge. In addition the roots are more flared to allow for the growth of a permanent tooth beneath it. This makes the cervix appear more constricted.

The crown has less enamel and the pulp horns extend more occlusally than they do in a permanent tooth. Because there is less enamel, the pulp is closer to the surface. Thus, care must be taken when engine polishing to avoid excessive friction. This heat could cause injury to the tooth. When one is familiar with permanent tooth structure it is easy to recognize the deciduous tooth that bears a close resemblance to it.

DESCRIPTION OF DECIDUOUS TEETH

Maxillary Teeth

Incisors. The labial crown of the incisor is smooth with a straight incisal edge; there are no mamelons. The crown is wide with a cingulum and marginal ridges on the lingual.

Canine. The cervical ridge of the canine is wide causing the cervix to appear constricted. The cusp tip is pointed, but short; the root is long and slender, Figure 13-3.

First Molar. The number of cusps can be 2, 3, or 4. There is no groove on the buccal surface to divide the cusps.

The occlusal surface has a central fossa and a mesial triangular fossa connected by a central groove. There are three roots, as with all maxillary molars, but the bifurcation of the buccal roots begins almost apically to the cervix.

Second Molar. The anatomy is the same as the permanent maxillary first molar, Figure 13-4. There are two buccal cusps divided by a buccal groove and two lingual cusps with a cusp of Carabelli, or fifth cusp groove, on the mesio-lingual cusp. There are three roots: two buccal, one lingual.

Mandibular Teeth

Incisors. Both labial and lingual surfaces are smooth although there is a cingulum and marginal ridges on the lingual.

Canines. The buccal has a pronounced cervical ridge. The lingual surface shows evidence of a cingulum and lingual ridges.

First Molar. As with the maxillary first molar, there is no definite anatomy. Usually there are two buccal cusps divided by a depression, rather than a groove, and two lingual cusps. There are two roots; both are long, slender, and divergent. The occlusal surface has a central groove crossed by the buccal groove and a lingual groove.

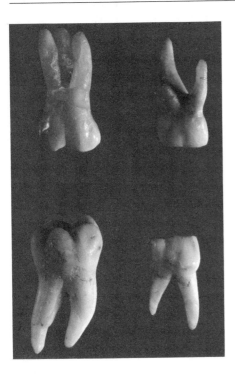

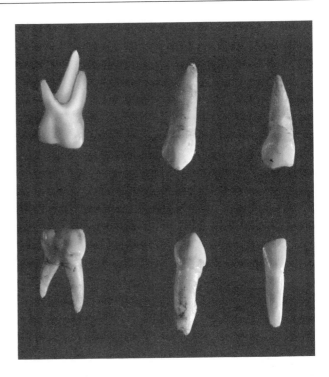

Figure 13-4 Deciduous molars compared to permanent molars

Figure 13-5 Deciduous incisors, canines, and molars

Second Molar. The anatomy is the same as that of the permanent mandibular first molar. Grooves divide the three buccal cusps and the two lingual cusps. The occlusal groove pattern is also the same as that on the permanent mandibular first molar although there may be more supplemental grooves. There are two long, thin, divergent roots which can be twice as long as the crown.

IMPORTANCE OF DECIDUOUS TEETH

The importance of the deciduous dentition must be realized, Figure 13-5. Each tooth has the same function as the permanent tooth which succeeds it. The deciduous teeth maintain a position for each permanent tooth replacement. If prematurely lost, the permanent replacement may erupt too early or emerge in an incorrect position. This sets the alignment for a future malocclusion or for periodontal problems. Because of these factors, it is important to stress care and maintenance of the deciduous teeth with the patient. The deciduous molar must be in a condition to function for about 10-12 years. Good dental habits developed during the early years will result in good maintenance of the permanent dentition.

SUMMARY

The deciduous dentition includes 10 maxillary and 10 mandibular teeth. Eruption begins around the 6th month of life and is completed between 2½ to 3 years. Each deciduous tooth resembles its succeeding permanent tooth, but is proportionately smaller. The posterior teeth have flared roots that allow for concurrent growth of the permanent teeth growing directly below.

Each deciduous tooth is an important part of the dentition, and it has a necessary function. It is important that they are cared for so that they endure until their natural exfoliation.

WORKSHEET

A. *Review the eruption sequence of the deciduous teeth.*
   List them in the correct sequence.

B. Using part A of the figure below, differentiate the molars.

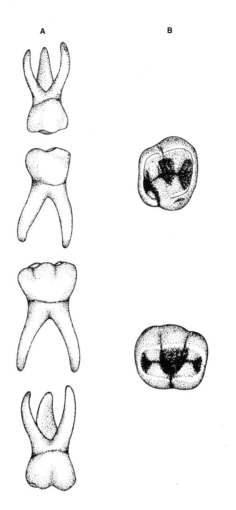

A   B

C. Using part B of the figure above, label the groove patterns of the deciduous second molars.

14

Tooth Development

INTRODUCTION
GROWTH AND DEVELOPMENT
ERUPTION
DEVELOPMENTAL ANOMALIES

Objectives

- Describe the development of the tooth during the following stages: growth (initiation, proliferation, histodifferentiation, and morphodifferentiation), apposition, and calcification.
- Define: active and passive eruption, proliferation, histodifferentiation, morphodifferentiation, apposition, supernumerary, and anomaly.
- Complete the worksheet at the end of the chapter.

INTRODUCTION

The development of a human begins with an embryo which has three layers: the ectoderm, the mesoderm, and the endoderm. The ectoderm will form not only the outer covering of the body, but the lining of the oral cavity. The skeletal and muscular systems, as well as other structures including the cementum, dentin, and pulp of the tooth form from the mesoderm. The lining of the internal organs develops from the endoderm.

During the third week of intrauterine life, when the embryo is only 3 mm long, the face begins its development. At one end of the embryo there is an invagination of the ectoderm forming the stomodeum, or primitive mouth, which later becomes the oral and nasal cavities.

The primitive mouth is lined with ectoderm and becomes the oral epithelium. Beneath this is the mesenchyme, developed from mesoderm, which becomes the underlying connective tissue.

Between the fifth and sixth week in utero, the first sign of tooth development is evident. Teeth are formed from the ectoderm and mesoderm in a complex histological process simplified into the following pattern.

GROWTH AND DEVELOPMENT

The growth stage is defined by an increase in the number and size of the cells, Figure 14-1. The formation of the teeth is a progression that begins during the fifth or sixth week in utero with the formation of the mandibular anterior teeth, followed shortly by the development of the maxillary anterior teeth. This developmental process continues, posteriorly, until 10 maxillary and 10 mandibular teeth are formed. The growth pattern is shown in Chapter 1, Figure 1-4. Permanent teeth begin forming about the fourth or fifth month of fetal life but do not calcify until after birth.

Initiation

Tooth development is initiated (started) with the formation of a tooth germ which produces the tissues of the tooth. Often, this is referred to as the "bud stage" of development because of a narrow band of oral epithelium, the primary dental lamina, which thickens and grows downward into the underlying tissue, resembling a bud. This process continues, posteriorly, until all the deciduous tooth buds are formed in each jaw.

Proliferation

A group of epithelial cells called the enamel organ is the first to form. This will produce the enamel of the tooth. These cells *proliferate,* or multiply at a rapid rate, and assume the shape of a cap. Within the cap is connective tissue arising from the mesoderm; this becomes the dental papilla which will make up the dentin and pulp of the tooth. Embodying the papilla is a fibrous dental sac, formed from mesoderm, that will become the periodontal ligament, cementum, and alveolar process.

Histodifferentiation

As the cells increase in number, they layer into the shape of a bell. Later, these cells become specialized, or differentiate into specialized tissues — ameloblasts, which form enamel, and odontoblasts, which form dentin. Separating these two cell layers is a basement membrane.

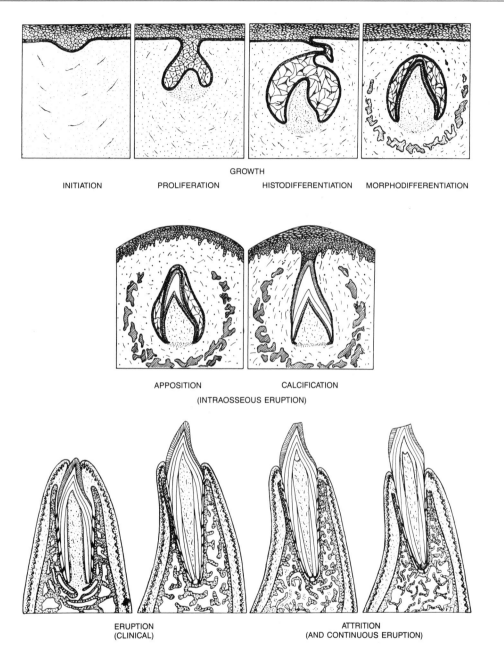

GROWTH

INITIATION   PROLIFERATION   HISTODIFFERENTIATION   MORPHODIFFERENTIATION

APPOSITION   CALCIFICATION

(INTRAOSSEOUS ERUPTION)

ERUPTION
(CLINICAL)

ATTRITION
(AND CONTINUOUS ERUPTION)

Figure 14-1 Life cycle of the tooth (Copyright by the American Dental Association. Reprinted by permission.)

Morphodifferentiation

While the tooth germ is developing, the surrounding area of the jaw also continues to develop. The bone cells will form the mandible and maxilla; the nerves and blood vessels will later be enveloped within the bone and teeth; and the tooth germ will assume the shape of a crown and root.

Around the fifth month of fetal development, the hard tissues of the tooth start to form. The dentin composition starts first, followed shortly by the enamel.

Apposition

During the final stage of tooth formation, the enamel and dentin increase in layers (*apposition*), until the tooth is completely shaped. As the tooth develops, its shaping begins at the incisal edge and progresses apically, in layers, until the crown, and then the roots are formed. However, keep in mind that eruption of the tooth occurs when only a portion of the root is formed. It will be several more years, after eruption, before the entire root is complete.

Calcification

Once the enamel and dentin have formed, the tooth matrix calcifies. The dentinal matrix calcifies progressively as it is produced, with each successive layer calcifying after the previous layer is laid down. The mineralization process of enamel is less clear. Research continues in order to clarify the many theories of how enamel calcifies.

Once the initial development of enamel occurs, it is no longer produced. On the other hand, the innermost layers of dentin can be produced at any age to form secondary dentin. Further clarification of this is available in oral histology textbooks.

ERUPTION

Eruption is the movement of the tooth from its position within the jaw to its position in the oral cavity. The process is divided into active and passive eruption.

Active Eruption

This is the process whereby the crown of the tooth first moves from within the jaw into the oral cavity, a process that continues until the tooth meets its antagonist in the opposite jaw. Active eruption begins when the crown of the tooth is complete and a portion of the root has started to form. When the tooth emerges into the oral cavity, only a portion of the root has formed, as previously described.

It will take 1½ to 3 years for the completion of a deciduous root and about 3 years after eruption for the completion of a permanent root. The entire process of permanent tooth development, from initiation to completion, takes about 10 years.

By the time a primary tooth erupts, its succedaneous replacement, the permanent tooth, has begun forming. With the exception of the permanent molars, this occurs beneath the root(s) of the deciduous tooth. Again, refer to the chart on tooth development in Chapter 1 for a review of the growth rate of teeth. Note that the first permanent molars begin calcifying after birth and develop in the area posterior to the second deciduous molars.

Passive Eruption

Once active eruption is complete, other factors that occur during life, such as wear from use or trauma, can cause attrition or breakdown of the periodontium. In turn, there can be exposure of cementum, wearing of the enamel, or gingival recession. This increase in the length of the clinical crown is referred to as passive eruption.

DEVELOPMENTAL ANOMALIES

Disturbances in the development stage of the teeth and bones can cause abnormalities. Hereditary or nutritional factors, such as excessive amounts of fluoride, may cause an *anomaly*, or deviation in the development of the teeth.

For example, any disturbance or interference in the fusion of the right and left maxillary process can result in a cleft of the palate. Disturbances during the formation of the tooth structure can cause faulty enamel or alteration of the shape of the tooth. Examples of this are enamel dysplasia, fluorosis, or peg-shaped lateral incisors. Occasionally, there may be an extra tooth that has formed called a *supernumerary* tooth. It is helpful to review the literature detailing the explanation of the causes of various tooth abnormalities in order to more clearly understand when and how these deviations occur.

SUMMARY

Between the fifth and sixth week in-utero, there is evidence of tooth development. An increase in growth and development of the cells continues until the entire tooth is formed, a process that lasts 2-3 years for the deciduous teeth and 9-10 years for the permanent teeth. Once a tooth is formed, it cannot repair itself like bones or skin. It is necessary to provide a proper diet during tooth formation and preventive care after eruption so that they last a lifetime.

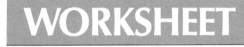

WORKSHEET

A. *Arrange the pictures in the correct chronological sequence and describe what occurs in each stage of development.*

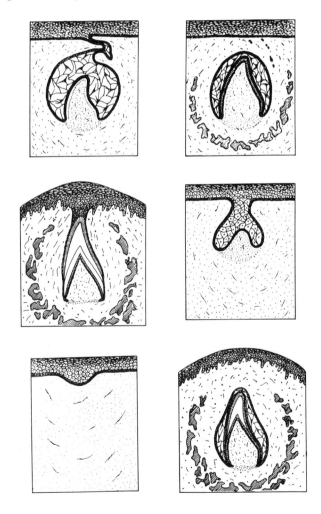

15

Occlusion

OCCLUSION
IDEAL OCCLUSION
NORMAL OCCLUSION
MALOCCLUSION
OCCLUSAL DEVIATIONS
ANGLE'S CLASSIFICATION OF OCCLUSION
RELATED TERMS
SPACING OF DECIDUOUS TEETH

Objectives

- Describe Angle's classification of occlusion.
- Describe five occlusal deviations that affect a group of teeth and explain the importance of deciduous teeth spacing on the occlusion of permanent teeth.
- List and explain five deviations of individual tooth positioning.
- Describe three types of facial profiles.
- Define the following terms: ideal occlusion, normal occlusion, malocclusion, centric occlusion, centric relation, terminal mesial step, terminal plane, and primate spacing.
- Complete the worksheet at the end of the chapter.

OCCLUSION

Occlusion occurs when the maxillary and mandibular teeth contact each other in any functional relationship. The study of occlusion is concerned with all the factors involved in the development, stability, and function of the *masticatory system*, not only with the contacting of the teeth. The masticatory system includes the teeth and surrounding structures, jaws, temporomandibular joint (TMJ), muscles, lips, tongue, and related nerves and blood vessels. Thus, the study of occlusion can be complex, extending beyond the arrangement of the teeth to include areas such as growth and development of the entire masticatory system, i.e. genetic as well as environmental factors.

Occlusion first occurs after the eruption of the deciduous dentition. The sequence of eruption, spacing, and positioning of the teeth, and the relationship of the jaws can be critical to occlusion, particularly if they vary significantly from the normal. The final occlusal relationship of the permanent dentition is a result of the influence of hereditary and environmental factors such as trauma, oral habits, or faulty dental treatment.

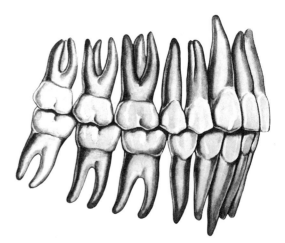

Figure 15-1 Permanent teeth in occlusion (Copyright by the American Dental Association. Reprinted by permission.)

IDEAL OCCLUSION

Ideal occlusion implies a complete, harmonious relationship of the teeth, as well as all other structures involved in the masticatory system, Figure 15-1. In an ideal anatomical occlusal relationship, the teeth conform to a specific pattern which includes 138 occlusal contacts in the closure of the 32 permanent teeth (Ramfjord & Ash, 1982). This ideal relationship, however, rarely exists.

When the maxillary and mandibular teeth are in an ideal position, the maxillary teeth facially overlap the mandibular teeth by one third, and each maxillary tooth has a distal relationship to its mandibular counterpart by the distance of about one half a tooth. Lingual cusps of maxillary posterior teeth occlude in specific fossae of mandibular teeth. An intercusp relationship such as this is referred to as *interdigitation*.

Ideal occlusion is noted, also, by the positioning of the permanent first molars and canines. The mesio-buccal cusp of the maxillary first molar will be positioned in the mesio-buccal groove of the mandibular first molar. The maxillary canine will occlude with the distal inclined plane on the marginal ridge of the mandibular canine and the mandibular first premolar.

NORMAL OCCLUSION

Since ideal occlusion seldom occurs, normal occlusion conforms closely to an ideal occlusal relationship but considers some variations from it. With normal occlusion, variations are considered optimum if there is functional comfort and stability of alignment. Normal or optimum occlusion is needed to maintain or protect the periodontium and/or TMJ, as well as for stabilization of alignment and aesthetics.

It is necessary that each tooth be able to withstand the forces exerted during mastication. The biting force of the posterior teeth is about 100-170 pounds. According to Phillips in *Elements of Dental Materials*, this represents 28,000 pounds per square inch or 300 pounds of pressure exerted by pressing down on a point with a medium sharp pencil. In proper occlusion, each tooth has an appropriate opposing contact. A malpositioned tooth can cause improper distribution of stress resulting in a breakdown of the periodontium and/or TMJ pathology.

According to Dr. Edward Angle, in a normal relationship, the first permanent molars are considered the key to occlusion and their position is the same as in ideal occlusion: the mesio-buccal cusp of the maxillary first molar rests in the mesio-buccal groove of the mandibular first molar.

MALOCCLUSION

Any deviation from ideal positioning of the teeth, whether it is a minor deviation of one tooth or a severe variation involving several teeth, or the jaws, creates a malocclusion. The best known system for classifying malocclusions was first described by Dr. Edward Angle in 1898. His system is based on the mesio-distal relationship of the maxillary and mandibular first molars and canines to each other — the maxillary first molar being his "key" to occlusion. Any variation in this relationship constitutes a malocclusion.

OCCLUSAL DEVIATIONS

Malocclusion or malalignment can affect an individual tooth or several teeth. Those involving several teeth are:

- **Openbite**—an existing space between the mandibular and maxillary teeth, Figure 15-2A. An openbite can be
    a. Anterior
    b. Posterior—unilateral or bilateral

- **Overbite**—a deep or vertical overlap of the maxillary teeth onto the mandibular teeth which exceeds the normal, or one-third depth of the mandibular incisors, Figure 15-2B.

- **Overjet**—a horizontal overlap creating a protrusion or space between the labial surface of the mandibular incisors and the lingual surface of the maxillary incisors, Figure 15-2C.

- **Crossbite**—a facially positioned mandibular tooth, or teeth. This can be
    a. Anterior
    b. Posterior—buccal or lingual, Figure 15-2D.

- **Edge-to-edge** or **end-to-end**—a contacting of the incisal edges or cusp tips rather than an interdigitation of cusp and fossae. Actually, this is a crossbite or precrossbite condition, Figure 15-2E.

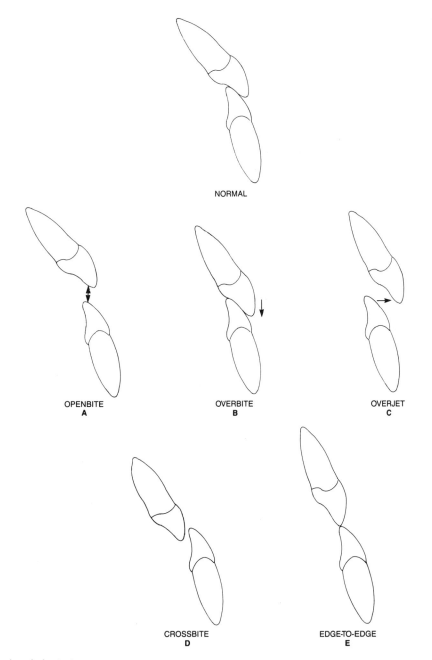

NORMAL

OPENBITE
A

OVERBITE
B

OVERJET
C

CROSSBITE
D

EDGE-TO-EDGE
E

Figure 15-2 Occlusal deviations

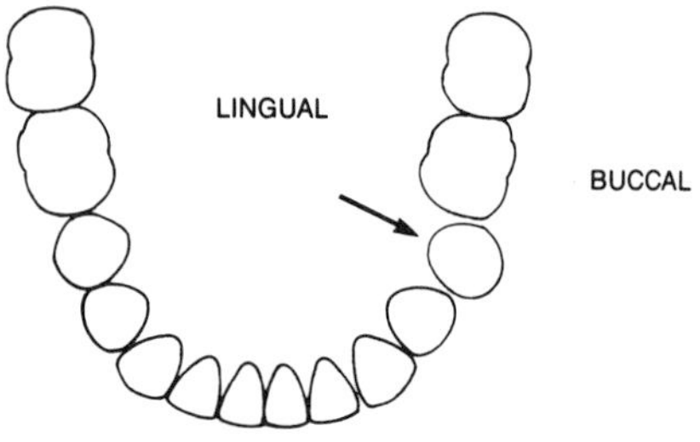

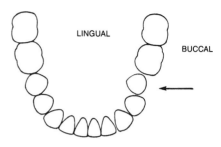

Figure 15-3 Buccoversion

Figure 15-4 Linguoversion

Those involving individual teeth are:

- **Labioversion** or **buccoversion**—a tooth positioned more facially than normal, Figure 15-3.

- **Linguoversion**—a tooth positioned more lingually than normal, Figure 15-4.

- **Infraversion**—a tooth positioned below the plane of occlusion, Figure 15-5.

- **Supraversion**—a tooth positioned above the plane of occlusion, Figure 15-6.

- **Torsoversion**—a rotated tooth, Figure 15-7.

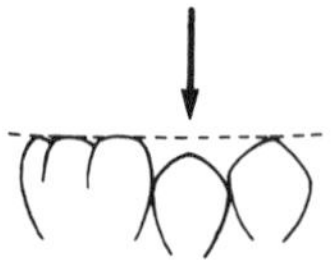

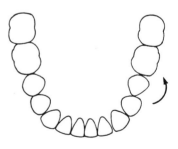

Figure 15-5 Infraversion

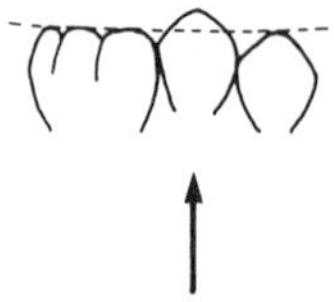

Figure 15-6 Supraversion

Figure 15-7 Torsoversion

ANGLE'S CLASSIFICATION OF OCCLUSION

Dr. Edward Angle was the first to develop a system to classify malocclusion. Since the mandible is movable, the classification relates to the anterior-posterior or mesio-distal deviations in relation to the first molar. There are three classifications (see Figure 15-8):

Class I—Neutro Occlusion (normal)

Both the permanent first molar and canine relationship are in ideal position. The mesio-buccal cusp of the maxillary first molar rests in the mesio-buccal groove of the mandibular first molar and the maxillary canine occludes with the distal inclined plane of the mandibular canine and the mandibular first premolar.

In a Class I relationship there can be deviations of a single or several anterior teeth such as an overjet or overbite, but the molars will have ideal positioning.

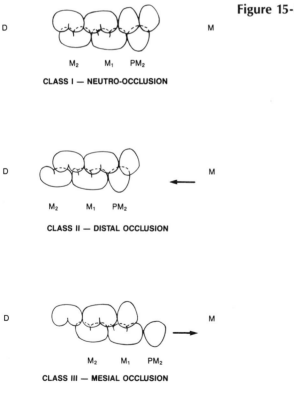

Figure 15-8 Angle's Classification of Occlusion

Class II—Distal Occlusion

The mandibular first permanent molar and canine are distal, or more posterior, by the width of a premolar, than the ideal position. Even when the molars are in a more distal position, other deviations can occur creating two divisions within a Class II occlusion:

Division I. A protrusion of incisors or overjet; overbite, crowding, or a labial inclination of the maxillary incisors.

Division II. A protrusion of the maxillary lateral incisors; a retrusion of the maxillary central incisors.

A Class II malocclusion can occur on one side of the arch while the other side remains a Class I. This is known as a *subdivision*; for example, Class II, Division I, Subdivision I.

Class III—Mesial Occlusion

The permanent mandibular first molar and canine are mesial, or more anterior, by the width of a premolar, than the normal position. When the molars are more mesially located, there are other conditions that can also occur such as an anterior crossbite or edge-to-edge contact of the anterior teeth.

Although it was developed almost 100 years ago, Angle's classification remains the most popular method of classifying malocclusions today. However, this classification is based solely on clinical examination. With the development of other techniques to diagnose true malocclusions, principally that of cephalometric radiographs and analyses, today's definitions of malocclusions go far beyond the relationship of maxillary and mandibular teeth to each other. These include the mesio-distal and anterior-posterior relationship of the mandible and maxilla to each other and to some fixed reference point, namely, the cranial bone. Today, the classification of malocclusion is more complicated as it considers not only dental anomalies but also skeletal and developmental deviations together with soft tissue and nasal and oral airway influences.

RELATED TERMS

Profiles: Mesiognathic is a normal profile, Figure 15-9A. When the mandible protrudes it is called prognathic (Figure 15-9B); when the mandible retrudes it is called retrognathic (Figure 15-9C).

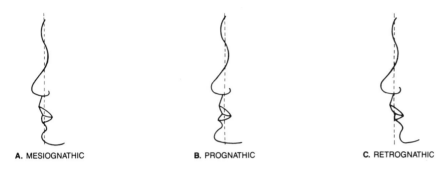

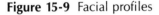

A. MESIOGNATHIC   B. PROGNATHIC   C. RETROGNATHIC

Figure 15-9 Facial profiles

Centric Occlusion: The relationship of the occlusal surfaces of one arch to those in the opposing arch at physical rest position. The posterior teeth are closed; the anterior teeth have very light or no contact.

Centric Relation: The most retruded position of the condyle in the mandibular fossa.

Mastication: The process whereby food is chewed. Food is chewed first on one side of the mouth and then shifted to the other side. The posterior teeth, with assistance of the cheeks, tongue and lips, perform the major portion of this work.

Functional Malocclusion: An occlusal deviation created by habits or muscular dysfunctions. Certain habits like thumbsucking or reverse swallowing may cause a malocclusion depending on the intensity, duration, and/or the age at which they occur.

Missing Teeth: Premature loss of deciduous teeth, missing permanent teeth or supernumerary teeth can also contribute to a malocclusion because they cause adjacent teeth to shift from their normal alignment.

SPACING OF DECIDUOUS TEETH

The spacing of the deciduous teeth plays an important part in the occlusion of the permanent teeth. Proximal contact is needed for the overall integrity of the permanent teeth but spacing between deciduous teeth, particularly the anterior teeth, is needed to provide adequate room for larger permanent teeth. This normal spacing between the anterior deciduous teeth is called *primate* spacing.

Although the jaws will grow, the growth may not provide enough width for the permanent teeth. Lack of primate spacing, or crowding of the anterior teeth, may suggest a future orthodontic problem.

The position of the deciduous second molar is also an important determinant of permanent tooth alignment. If the second molars are in a Class I position, the permanent teeth will usually be guided into a Class I position. The positioning of the deciduous second molars is then referred to as *Class I—terminal mesial step*, Figure 15-10A.

Often, the deciduous molars will show a cusp-to-cusp (end-to-end) relationship called *terminal plane*, Figure 15-10B. An actual end-to-end relationship between the second deciduous molars is also considered a Class I. If the deciduous molars guide the permanent molars into position, it appears as if this could lead to a malocclusion but often it does not. Extra space is provided in the area of the deciduous molars allowing for a mesial shift of the permanent mandibular first molars. The deciduous second molars are wider mesio-distally than the premolars that will replace them and there is a primate space between the deciduous canine and first molar. With these two factors and more growth in the arch between ages eight and nine, a Class I can occur.

SUMMARY

Occlusion occurs when the maxillary and mandibular teeth are in contact in any functional relationship. Ideal occlusion occurs when the teeth conform to a specific pattern of contacts. To simplify the study of occlusion, Angle's classification is frequently used to describe the relationship of first molars and canines. Deviations in position of teeth or groups of teeth provide a basic understanding of

Figure 15-10 Positioning of deciduous second molars

A. CLASS I — TERMINAL MESIAL STEP

B. TERMINAL PLANE

occlusion, but a thorough study of this subject would include all the factors involved in the development, stability, and function of the masticatory system.

WORKSHEET

A. *Using the following illustrations of the maxillary incisor as a guide, draw the mandibular incisor in the appropriate position as labeled.*

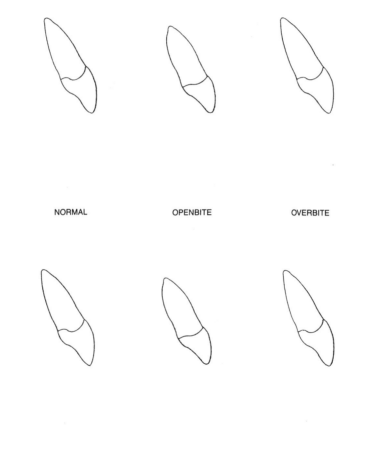

NORMAL	OPENBITE	OVERBITE

OVERJET	CROSSBITE	EDGE-TO-EDGE

B. *Using the following drawing of the mandibular arch, draw the premolar in the positions that are labeled.*

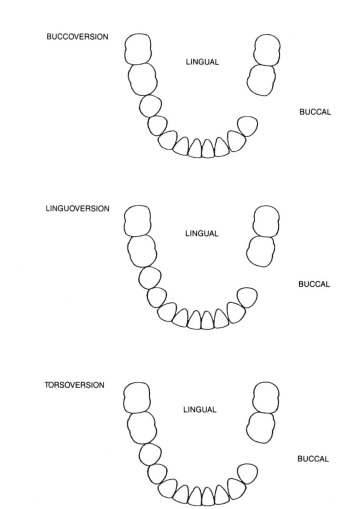

C. *Position the mandibular molar correctly into the following drawings, as labeled.*

MAXILLARY ARCH

NEUTRO-OCCLUSION

MAXILLARY ARCH

DISTAL OCCLUSION

MAXILLARY ARCH

MESIAL OCCLUSION

16

Form and Function

PROXIMAL CONTACT AREAS
INTERPROXIMAL SPACES
EMBRASURES
COMPENSATING CURVATURES

Objectives

- Describe proximal contact areas, interproximal spaces, and embrasures and give their importance to the function and integrity of the masticatory system.
- Define Curve of Spee and Curve of Wilson.
- Complete the worksheet at the end of the chapter.

In order for the teeth to cut and masticate food, their appropriate position in the arch must be maintained. Correct positioning is also necessary to assist in the protection of the supporting structures which in turn sustain the teeth so that they can function properly. Form and function are concerned with how both the position and shape of the teeth enable them to function.

The entire topic of tooth form and function is considerably broad, covering all the conditions that affect tooth alignment in the arches. *Wheeler's Dental Anatomy, Physiology and Occlusion*, by M. Ash, includes nine aspects in the study of this topic:

1. The development of occlusion.
2. Dental arch form.
3. Compensating curvatures and planes of the dental arches.
4. Angulation of the individual teeth in relation to various planes.

5. Functional form of the teeth at their incisal and occlusal thirds.

6. Facial relations of each tooth in one arch to its antagonist(s) in the opposing arch in centric occlusion.

7. Occlusal contact and intercusp relations of all teeth of one arch with those in the opposing arch in centric occlusion.

8. Occlusal contact and intercusp relations of all teeth during various functional mandibular movement.

9. Neurobehavioral aspects of occlusion.

An entire study of occlusion would be necessary to thoroughly cover these topics. Only a basic introduction to form and function is given in this chapter, covering those aspects that are most useful to a dental auxiliary. This includes the topics of proximal contact areas, interproximal space, and embrasures. Further study is recommended when considering oromotor functions, prosthetic rehabilitation, or orthodontics.

PROXIMAL CONTACT AREAS

The proximal contact area is a small spot on the mesial and distal surface of each tooth that touches, or contacts, the proximal tooth. Every tooth, except the last molars in each arch, has both a distal and mesial contact area. Contact areas are shown on Figure 16-1 by horizontal lines. This area is generally the widest point on the crown of the tooth.

Contact areas of anterior teeth are located more incisally than those of the posterior teeth. A review of the individual teeth shows the contact areas of the posterior teeth located about in the middle of the tooth.

Function of Contact Areas

Proper contact between teeth prevents food from packing between them. This, then, protects the gingiva from any irritation that could result from food that is lodged between the teeth. In addition, contact areas stabilize the teeth in the arch by providing mutual support.

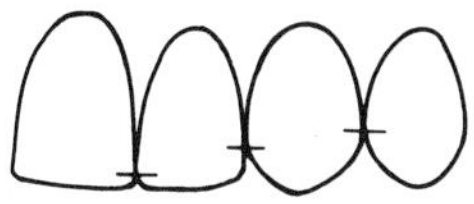

Figure 16-1 Contact areas

INTERPROXIMAL SPACES

The interproximal space is an area between each tooth normally filled with the interdental papilla. Its boundaries form a triangle with the sides as the proximal surfaces of the teeth; the base is the alveolar crest and the apex is the contact area, Figure 16-2.

Function of the Interproximal Space

Appropriate width between each tooth (the base of the triangle) is important to provide enough space for periodontal structures; to allow ample bone between each tooth for adequate support; and to maintain the level of the gingival tissue.

EMBRASURES

Any curvature, either toward or away from the contact area, is an embrasure, Figure 16-3. Embrasures are located on the incisal, occlusal, lingual, or facial surface and are often referred to as spillways because they assist the food in "spilling" away from the tooth.

Figure 16-2 The boundaries of the interproximal form a triangle.

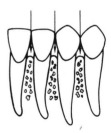

INTERPROXIMAL SPACES

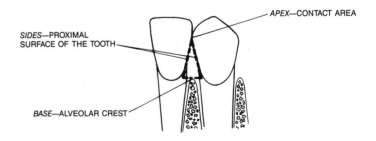

APEX—CONTACT AREA

SIDES—PROXIMAL SURFACE OF THE TOOTH

BASE—ALVEOLAR CREST

Function of the Embrasures

The embrasures or spillways act as an escapement for food so that it does not cling to the teeth or get forced into the interproximal spaces. In this way, embrasures act to assist in cleansing the tooth and to protect the gingival tissue from being irritated by keeping the food away from it.

COMPENSATING CURVATURES

The occlusal plane of the tooth is a line that extends from the incisal edge of the central incisors to the distal buccal cusp of the second molar. Von Spee first noted that this line, when viewed from a point opposite the first molars, forms a curve when the teeth have erupted and are in normal alignment. This curve, which is concave toward the mandible, is the Curve of Spee, named after Von Spee, who first defined it, Figure 16-4.

OCCLUSAL EMBRASURE

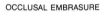

FACIAL VIEW

LINGUAL EMBRASURE

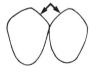

FACIAL EMBRASURE

OCCLUSAL VIEW

Figure 16-3 Embrasures

CURVE OF SPEE

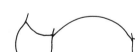

FACIAL VIEW

CURVE OF WILSON

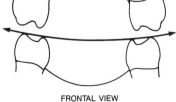

FRONTAL VIEW

Figure 16-4 The Curve of Spee and the Curve of Wilson—frontal views

When the arches are viewed from a frontal position, another curvature is seen extending from the cusp tip of the right molar to the cusp tip of the left molar. This concave curvature is the Curve of Wilson (see Figure 16-4).

Together, these and other compensating curvatures of the arches account for strength and efficiency in mastication and assist in the stability of the teeth. Compensating curvatures have no special use other than to help define occlusion. Their main use would be in the construction of dentures or in the balancing of the arches for orthodontia.

SUMMARY

Although there are many factors that affect the form and function of the teeth, three of these are examined in order to provide a basic understanding of the importance of the appropriate positioning of each tooth in the arch. Those examined are: proper proximal contact areas, which prevent food from packing between the teeth; embrasures, which act as a spillway so that food does not cling to the teeth; and interproximal spacing, which allows adequate space for the periodontal structures to support the teeth.

WORKSHEET

A. *Complete the following questions about contact areas.*

1. Tooth surfaces that are adjacent to, or facing each other are called prox-

    imal surfaces. The proximal surfaces are the _____ and

    _____ surfaces of each tooth.

2. The contact area is that *area* of the proximal surface that touches the adjacent area. Each tooth contacts its adjacent tooth on the proximal surface.

    Each tooth has two contact areas except the last molar which has no contacting tooth on the distal.

    Mesial surfaces contact distal surfaces with the exception of the central incisors where two mesial surfaces meet.

Place a line on the following figure to represent the location of the contact areas.

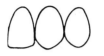

B. *Complete the following questions about interproximal space.*
Cervical to each contact area is the interproximal space. In the oral cavity the interproximal space is filled by the interdental papilla. The arrow in the figure below points to the interproximal space.

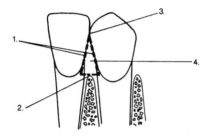

The boundaries of the interproximal space form a triangle.

The sides of the triangle are formed by _____ (1)

The base of the triangle is the _____ (2)

The apex of the triangle is the _____ (3)

The contact area is filled with gingiva called _____ (4)

C. *On the figure below, locate an embrasure and label it.*
Any curvature adjacent to the contact area is called an embrasure. This can be located on any surface of the tooth.

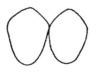   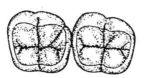

D. *Complete the following chart by putting an X in the appropriate square.*

	INTERPROXIMAL SPACE	CONTACT AREA	EMBRASURE
Stabilizes the Tooth			
Helps Tooth to be Self-Cleansing			
Protects the Gingiva			
Keeps Food from Packing between the Teeth			
Contains Interdental Papilla			

SECTION FIVE
HEAD AND NECK ANATOMY

17

Osteology of the Skull

NEUROCRANIUM
VISCEROCRANIUM
MAXILLA
MANDIBLE
HYOID BONE

Objectives

- Identify the location of the cranial and facial bones, noted in italics in the chapter.
- Identify the location of the anatomical landmarks on the cranial and facial bones.
- Identify the following foramina or canals: hypoglossal canal, supraorbital, stylomastoid, carotid canal, jugular, rotundum, ovale, foramen magnum, spinosum, lacerum, greater and lesser palantine, incisive.
- Identify the location of the anatomical landmarks on the mandible and maxilla, noted in italics in the chapter.
- Complete the worksheet at the end of this chapter.

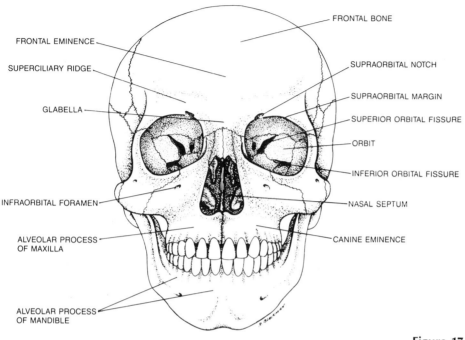

FRONTAL BONE
FRONTAL EMINENCE
SUPERCILIARY RIDGE
GLABELLA
INFRAORBITAL FORAMEN
ALVEOLAR PROCESS OF MAXILLA
ALVEOLAR PROCESS OF MANDIBLE
SUPRAORBITAL NOTCH
SUPRAORBITAL MARGIN
SUPERIOR ORBITAL FISSURE
ORBIT
INFERIOR ORBITAL FISSURE
NASAL SEPTUM
CANINE EMINENCE

Figure 17-1 Skull, anterior aspect

NEUROCRANIUM

There are 22 bones that make up the skull. The *neurocranium* is the portion of the cranium that houses and protects the brain. It is made up of the following eight bones (Figures 17-1 through 17-4):

Single Bones	Paired (Right and Left) Bones
Occipital	Parietal
Sphenoid	Temporal
Ethmoid	
Frontal	

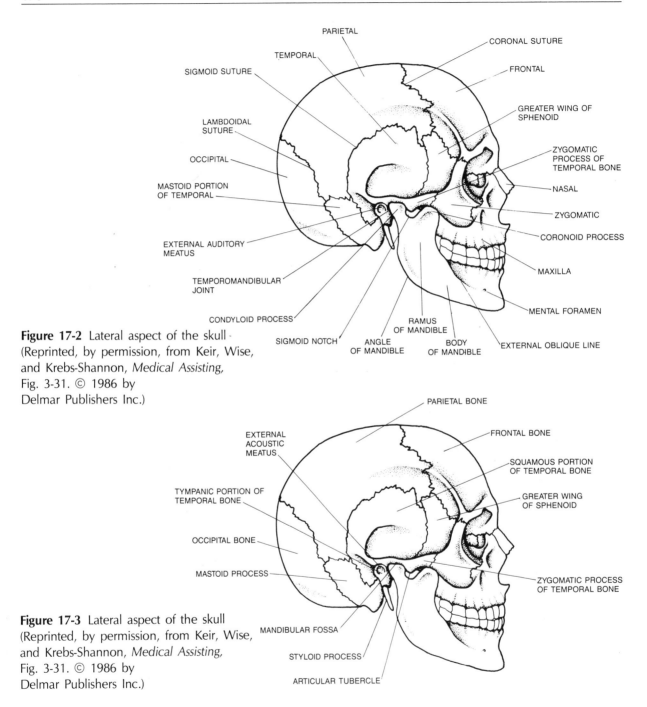

Figure 17-2 Lateral aspect of the skull (Reprinted, by permission, from Keir, Wise, and Krebs-Shannon, *Medical Assisting,* Fig. 3-31. © 1986 by Delmar Publishers Inc.)

Figure 17-3 Lateral aspect of the skull (Reprinted, by permission, from Keir, Wise, and Krebs-Shannon, *Medical Assisting,* Fig. 3-31. © 1986 by Delmar Publishers Inc.)

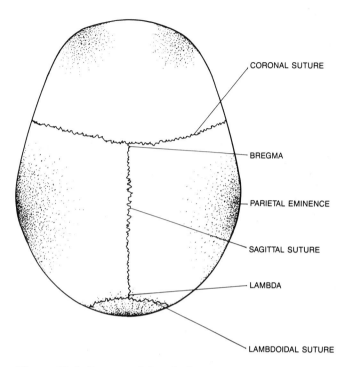

CORONAL SUTURE

BREGMA

PARIETAL EMINENCE

SAGITTAL SUTURE

LAMBDA

LAMBDOIDAL SUTURE

Figure 17-4 Sutures of the skull

This chapter introduces several new terms. A *suture* is a jagged line where bones join. A *foramen* is a short opening through bone, and a *canal* is a long opening through bone. Nerves and blood vessels travel through canals and foramina.

Occipital Bone

The occipital bone forms the posterior aspect of the skull. It articulates or joins with the atlas, or first cervical vertebra, by way of the *occipital condyles*. These condyles are located on either side of the *foramen magnum*, the large opening through which the spinal cord passes (Figure 17-5).

From an internal view, the occipital bone is divided into four fossae which house lobes of the brain. The *hypoglossal canals* are located on either side of the foramen magnum. The hypoglossal nerve, an important nerve in dentistry, passes through the hypoglossal canal (Figure 17-6).

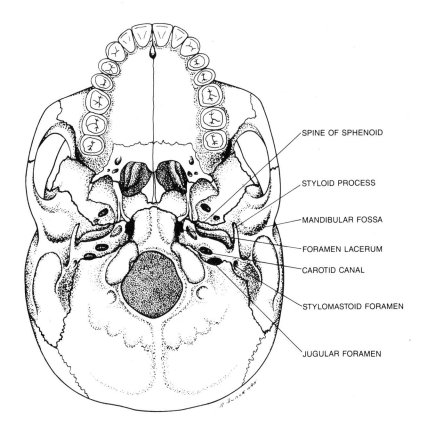

SPINE OF SPHENOID

STYLOID PROCESS

MANDIBULAR FOSSA

FORAMEN LACERUM

CAROTID CANAL

STYLOMASTOID FORAMEN

JUGULAR FORAMEN

Figure 17-5 Inferior aspect of the skull

Frontal Bone

This bone forms the forehead and anterior aspect of the skull (Figures 17-1 through 17-4). There are four sutures which outline or delineate this bone.

1. *Coronal suture* — joins the frontal and parietal bones

2. *Sagittal suture* — connects the parietal bones

3. *Lambdoidal suture* — joins the occipital and parietal bones

4. *Squamous suture* — connects the parietal and temporal bones

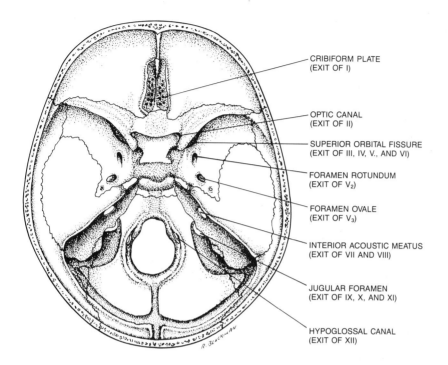

CRIBIFORM PLATE
(EXIT OF I)

OPTIC CANAL
(EXIT OF II)

SUPERIOR ORBITAL FISSURE
(EXIT OF III, IV, V., AND VI)

FORAMEN ROTUNDUM
(EXIT OF V_2)

FORAMEN OVALE
(EXIT OF V_3)

INTERIOR ACOUSTIC MEATUS
(EXIT OF VII AND VIII)

JUGULAR FORAMEN
(EXIT OF IX, X, AND XI)

HYPOGLOSSAL CANAL
(EXIT OF XII)

Figure 17-6 The skull, internal aspect, showing sites of exit of the cranial nerves

The *bregma* is the intersection between the coronal and sagittal sutures. The *lambda* is the intersection between the sagittal and lambdoidal sutures (Figure 17-4).

The prominent area of the forehead is known as the *frontal eminence*. The *glabella* is the flattened area between the eyebrows. A *superciliary ridge* is located above each eyebrow. On the superior margin of the orbit (eye) is the *supraorbital foramen* through which passes the supraorbital nerve and artery (Figure 17-1).

Bones of the Orbit

Six bones make up each orbit: sphenoid, ethmoid, lacrimal, frontal, zygomatic, and maxilla (Figures 17-1 and 17-7). The *optic foramen* is the opening for the optic nerve and ophthalmic artery. Through the *superior orbital fissure*, the oculomotor (III), trochlear (IV), ophthalmic branch of the trigeminal (V), and the abducent (VI) nerves enter the orbit. The *inferior orbital fissure* is the entrance to the orbit for the infraorbital nerve.

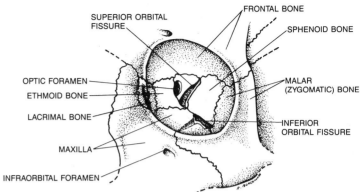

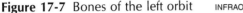

Figure 17-7 Bones of the left orbit

Parietal Bones

The parietal bones have two curving lines, the superior and inferior temporal lines (Figures 17-2 through 17-4). These lines serve as the attachment for the temporalis muscle, a muscle of mastication.

Temporal Bones

The temporal bones consist of three parts: the squamous, which is the flattened, fan-shaped portion; the petrous; and the tympanic which encloses the essential hearing organs (Figures 17-2, 17-3, and 17-5). The temporal bones have several portions:

- the *zygomatic process* extends out to form the zygomatic arch.
- the *mandibular (glenoid) fossa*, into which the mandible articulates.
- the *articular eminence* or *tubercle*, a V-shaped projection located in front of the glenoid fossa (Figure 17-2).

The *external auditory (acoustic) meatus*, located in the tympanic portion, is the opening for the outer ear. Posterior to this meatus is a rounded prominence known as the *mastoid process* (Figure 17-2). This structure is hollowed out by air cells that communicate with the middle ear. A pointed spicule of bone, the *styloid process*, serves as a muscle and ligament attachment. A small foramen, the *stylomastoid foramen*, is located between the styloid and mastoid processes. This is the opening through which the facial nerve (VII) exits the skull (Figure 17-5).

Just lateral to the occipital condyles and between the petrous portions of the temporal bone is the *jugular foramen*, a large opening, through which the internal jugular vein, glossopharyngeal (IV), vagus (X), and (spinal) accessory (XI) nerves exit the skull. The *carotid canal* opening for the internal carotid artery is located in front of the jugular foramen (Figure 17-5).

Ethmoid Bone

This bone forms a part of the nasal cavity, nasal septum, and the orbit. It is located anteriorly at the base of the cranium and is made up of a perpendicular or *cribiform plate*. The cribiform plate is perforated to allow olfactory nerves (smell) to pass between the brain and nose. The ethmoid bone can be a part of the neurocranium or viscerocranium. For our purposes, we will consider it a portion of the neurocranium.

Sphenoid Bone

This bone looks like a bat with a body, two greater wings and two lesser wings (Figures 17-6, 17-8, and 17-9). It articulates with *all* the bones that form the

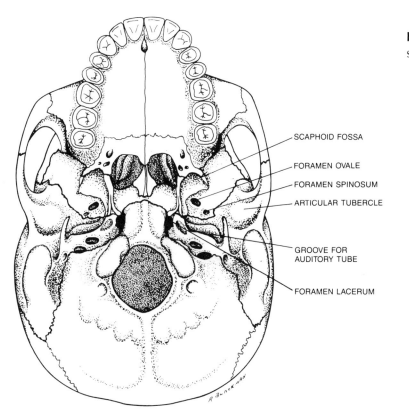

Figure 17-8 Skull: inferior aspect, showing foramina

SCAPHOID FOSSA

FORAMEN OVALE

FORAMEN SPINOSUM

ARTICULAR TUBERCLE

GROOVE FOR
AUDITORY TUBE

FORAMEN LACERUM

cranium. From each greater wing (like butterfly wings), a *pterygoid process* descends. Each pterygoid process (Figure 17-9) is made up of:

- flattened, lateral plate (outside)
- thinner, medial plate (inside)
- pterygoid (scaphoid) fossa — a depression between the medial and lateral plates
- pterygoid hamulus — a pointed process that curves outward from the lower (free) end of the medial plate

A depression seen on the surface of the sphenoid bone houses the *pituitary gland*. This depression is known as the *sella turcica* (Figure 17-9).

Three foramina can be seen on the sphenoid bone from the internal aspect. The *foramen rotundum* transmits the maxillary division of the trigeminal nerve (V_2). Through the *foramen ovale*, the mandibular division of the trigeminal nerve (V_3) passes. The *foramen spinosum* (Figure 17-8) transmits the middle meningeal artery to the brain. Next to the foramen ovale is the *foramen lacerum* (Figure 17-8), a channel through which the internal carotid artery travels. In a living human being, the foramen lacerum is covered by a layer of cartilage (Figures 17-5 and 17-6).

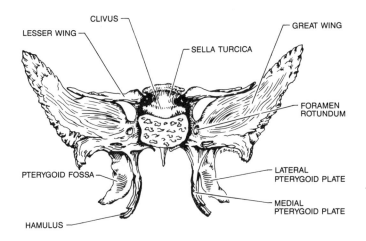

Figure 17-9 Sphenoid bone

VISCEROCRANIUM

There are fourteen bones that make up the viscerocranium of the facial skeleton which gives us our appearance.

Single Bones	Paired (Right and Left) Bones
Mandible	Zygomatic
Vomer	Maxillae
	Nasal
	Lacrimal
	Palatine
	Inferior nasal concha

Zygomatic Bones (Cheek Bones)

The zygomatic (sing. zygoma) bones form the cheeks.

Vomer

The vomer forms the posterior and inferior part of the nasal septum (Figure 17-11). The ethmoid bone forms the anterior portion of the nasal septum.

Nasal Bones

These oblong bones form the bridge of the nose (Figures 17-1 and 17-2).

Lacrimal Bones

The lacrimal bones are small and fragile (Figure 17-7). They are located at the anterior portion of the medial orbital wall.

Inferior Nasal Concha

The inferior nasal concha lies in the nasal cavity and articulates with the maxilla. The superior and middle nasal concha are processes of the ethmoid bone, however, the inferior nasal concha is formed as a separate bone (Figure 17-11).

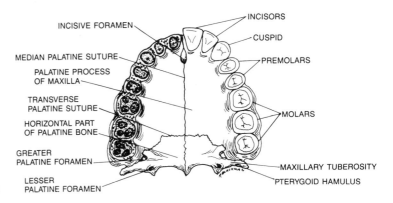

INCISIVE FORAMEN
INCISORS
CUSPID
MEDIAN PALATINE SUTURE
PREMOLARS
PALATINE PROCESS OF MAXILLA
TRANSVERSE PALATINE SUTURE
MOLARS
HORIZONTAL PART OF PALATINE BONE
GREATER PALATINE FORAMEN
MAXILLARY TUBEROSITY
LESSER PALATINE FORAMEN
PTERYGOID HAMULUS

Figure 17-10 Maxilla: bony palate

Palatine Bones

Each palatine bone is made up of a horizontal plate, which forms the hard palate, and a vertical plate. Two foramina are located in the hard palate. The *greater palatine foramen* is a large opening for the greater palatine nerve and artery. The *lesser palatine foramen* is a small foramen located posterior to the greater palatine foramen. It transmits the lesser palatine nerve and artery (Figure 17-10).

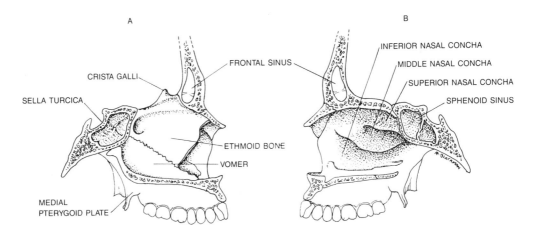

A
B
FRONTAL SINUS
INFERIOR NASAL CONCHA
CRISTA GALLI
MIDDLE NASAL CONCHA
SUPERIOR NASAL CONCHA
SELLA TURCICA
SPHENOID SINUS
ETHMOID BONE
VOMER
MEDIAL PTERYGOID PLATE

Figure 17-11 Bony nasal septum and cavity: (A) sagittal section showing the bony nasal septum, (B) nasal cavity with nasal septum removed

MAXILLA

The maxilla is made up of two portions joined by a median suture. It consists of a body and four processes. The *frontal process* and *zygomatic* (molar) *process* join the frontal and zygomatic bones. The *alveolar process* surrounds and supports the maxillary teeth and the *palatine process* forms the major portion of the hard palate.

The body of the maxilla contains the *canine eminence,* an elevation of bone over the canine root. The infraorbital nerve exits onto the face through the *infraorbital foramen* just below the inferior margin of the orbit (Figure 17-1). The *maxillary sinus* is the largest of the paranasal sinuses and is located within the maxilla above the roots of the maxillary posterior teeth. Posterior to the maxillary third molars is a bulging of bone known as the maxillary tuberosity (Figure 17-10).

From an interior view, the *incisive (nasopalatine) foramen* can be seen. It is located on the midline, just behind the maxillary central incisors. It is the opening for the nasopalatine nerve to innervate the hard palate in the maxillary anterior region. It is covered by the incisive papillae (Figure 17-10). The *median palatine suture* marks the articulation of the right and left palatine process. The *transverse palatine suture* is the articulation between the palatine process and the horizontal plates of the palatine bones.

MANDIBLE

This is a horseshoe-shaped bone that is made up of a horizontal *body* with a right and left vertical *rami* (sing. ramus). There is one body and two rami. Each rami has:

- a *condyle* — a rounded knob that joins with the mandibular (glenoid) fossa
- a *coronoid process* — a pointed, flat projection onto which the temporalis muscle inserts
- a *coronoid, mandibular* or *sigmoid notch* — the curved notch between the condyle and coronoid process (Figure 17-12)

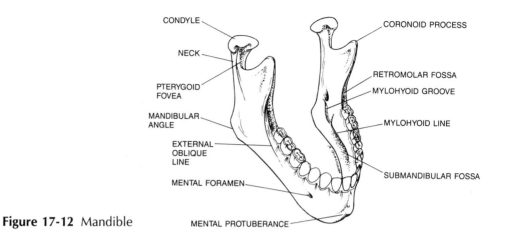

Figure 17-12 Mandible

The condyle is attached to the ramus by a thin neck. A triangular depression below the condyle is known as the *pterygoid fovea* to which the lateral pterygoid muscle attaches (Figure 17-12). The *mental protuberance* is the tip of the chin. The *mental foramen* is located on the external surface of the mandible near the apex of the mandibular second premolar. It is the exit point where the mental nerve and vessels branch from the inferior alveolar nerve. A line that extends from the mental foramen along the external surface of the body is known as the *external oblique line* (Figure 17-12).

Internal Surface. On the internal surface of the mandible, the *internal oblique line* can be seen. It runs from the molar region to the midline. It is also known as the *mylohyoid ridge* or *line* and is the attachment for the mylohyoid muscle. *Genial tubercles* or *spines,* small projections of bone located on either side of the midline (Figure 17-13), are the site of attachment for the genioglossus and geniohyoid muscles.

Figure 17-13 Mandible: posterior view

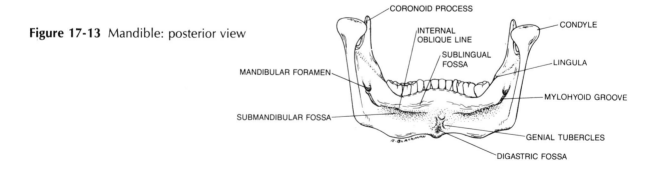

The *submandibular fossa* contains the submandibular gland, and is located in the premolar and molar region below the mylohyoid line. The sublingual fossa is located on either side of the genial tubercles. The sublingual glands are housed here (Figure 17-13).

The *retromolar fossa* is a triangular area of bone distal to the mandibular third molar (Figure 17-12). The *mandibular foramen* is a large opening located in the center of the ramus. It is the opening into the mandibular canal through which passes the inferior alveolar nerve and artery (Figures 17-12 and 17-13). Superior to the mandibular foramen is the *lingula,* a small bony projection which protects the foramen. The *mylohyoid groove* may be visible leading away from the mandibular foramen (Figure 17-13).

HYOID BONE

The hyoid bone is suspended in the neck and is an attachment point for neck and tongue muscles. It is made up of a body and two pairs of horns, the greater cornu and lesser cornu (Figure 17-14). It is horseshoe-shaped and does not articulate with other bones.

SUMMARY

The skeleton of the skull is divided into two groups: (1) the neurocranium, 22 bones that make up the skull and (2) the viscerocranium, 14 bones that make up the face.

Included in the neurocranium are (1) the occipital bone, which forms the posterior aspect of the skull; (2) the frontal bone, which forms the forehead and anterior aspect of the skull; (3) the ethmoid bone, which forms the nasal cavity, nasal septum, and orbit; (4) the sphenoid, ethmoid, lacrimal, frontal, zygomatic,

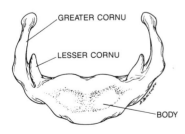

Figure 17-14 Hyoid bone: anterior view

and maxilla, which make up the bones of the orbit; (5) the parietal bones, which form the sides of the skull; and (6) the temporal bones, which house the hearing organs and help to make up the temporomandibular joint.

Included in the viscerocranium are (1) the zygomatic bones, which form the cheek; (2) the nasal bones, which form the bridge of the nose; (3) the lacrimal bones; (4) the inferior nasal concha, which lies in the nasal cavity and articulates with the maxilla; (5) the palatine bones, which form the hard palate; (6) the maxilla, which forms the upper jaw; (7) the mandible, which forms the lower jaw; and the vomer, which forms the posterior and inferior part of the nasal septum.

In addition, the hyoid bone, which does not articulate with other bones, is located in the skull. It serves as an attachment for the tongue and neck muscles.

WORKSHEET

A. Define the following terms.

> foramen
> canal
> suture

B. Using a human skull:

1. Locate the following bones:
   occipital
   frontal
   parietal
   temporal
   sphenoid
   ethmoid
   zygomatic
   nasal
   lacrimal
   inferior nasal concha
   palatine

2. Locate the following structures on the sphenoid bone.
    lateral plate
    medial plate
    pterygoid fossa
    pterygoid hamulus

3. Locate the following structures on the maxilla.
    canine eminence
    infraorbital foramen
    maxillary tuberosity
    incisive foramen
    median palatine suture
    transverse palatine suture
    greater palatine foramen
    lesser palatine foramen

4. Locate the following structures on the mandible.
    body
    ramus
    condyle
    coronoid process
    pterygoid fovea
    mental protuberance
    mental foramen
    external oblique line
    internal oblique line
    genial tubercles
    submandibular fossa
    sublingual fossa
    retromolar fossa
    mandibular foramen
    mylohyoid groove
    lingula

C. Complete the following figures.

1. Please name the structure indicated by each line. Just in case the line is not clear, the structures to be named are listed below.

   1. Frontal bone
   2. Mental protuberance
   3. Mental foramen
   4. Supraorbital notch or foramen
   5. Infraorbital foramen

   6. Superior orbital fissure
   7. Sphenoid bone
   8. Nasal bones
   9. Inferior orbital fissure
   10. Ramus mandible

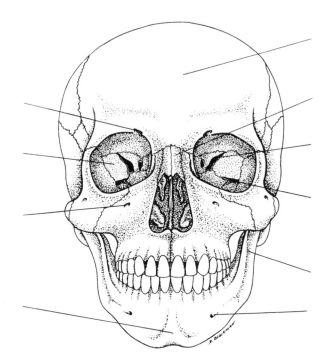

2. Please name the structures indicated by each line. Be certain to name all the structures listed below.

1. Medial pterygoid plate
2. Pterygoid hamulus
3. Lateral pterygoid plate
4. Pterygoid (scaphoid) fossa
5. Foramen magnum
6. Incisive foramen
7. Median palatine suture
8. Transverse palatine suture
9. Styloid process
10. Occipital condyle

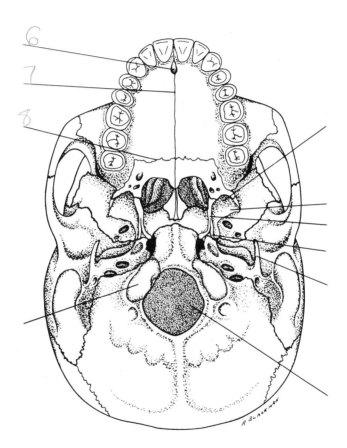

3. Please name the structures indicated by each line. Be certain to name all the structures from the list below.

1. Pterygoid fovea
2. Condyle
3. Coronoid process
4. Lingula
5. Mandibular foramen

6. Mylohyoid groove
7. Mylohyoid ridge or line
8. Coronoid notch (mandibular or sigmoid)
9. Retromolar triangle or fossa
10. Angle of the mandible

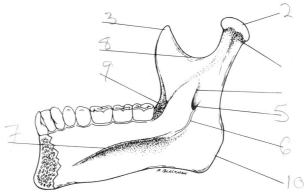

D. Answer the following questions.

1. Name the bones that make up the neurocranium.

2. Name the bones that make up the viscerocranium.

3. List the bones on which the following landmarks are located.
    a. foramen magnum
    b. glabella
    c. glenoid fossa
    d. sella turcica
    e. cribiform plate

4. What bone joins with all other cranial bones?

5. What bone does not join with any bones?

18

Muscles of the Head and Neck

MUSCLES OF MASTICATION
SUPRAHYOID MUSCLES
INFRAHYOID MUSCLES
MUSCLES OF THE TONGUE
MUSCLES OF FACIAL EXPRESSION
MUSCLES OF THE NECK
MUSCLES OF THE SOFT PALATE
MUSCLES OF THE PHARYNX

Objectives

- Describe the origin, insertion, and function of the muscles of mastication.
- Classify each muscle of the head and neck according to the group in which it belongs.
- Describe the location and function of the muscles of facial expression, suprahyoid and infrahyoid muscles, and muscles of the tongue, neck, soft palate, and pharynx.
- Describe nerve innervation to the various muscle groups.
- Describe the three stages of swallowing.
- Complete the worksheet at the end of the chapter.

Muscles make movements possible by their contraction. Generally, they are suspended between an *origin*, a fixed structure or end, and an *insertion*, the movable end. Names of the muscles may give their origin and insertion. Since muscles move in the direction of their origin, this helps in understanding their motion. The muscles of the head and neck are divided into eight groups:

- Muscles of mastication
- Suprahyoid muscles
- Infrahyoid muscles
- Muscles of the tongue
- Muscles of facial expression
- Muscles of the neck
- Muscles of the soft palate
- Muscles of the pharynx

MUSCLES OF MASTICATION

These muscles elevate, protrude, retrude, or cause lateral movement of the mandible. They work during chewing or *mastication*, hence their name. They are innervated by the mandibular branch of the trigeminal nerve (V_3). The maxillary artery provides blood supply.

Temporalis

The temporalis muscle is the most powerful muscle to elevate the jaw (Figure 18-1). This fan-shaped muscle starts from the temporal fossa of the temporal bone. The fibers form an anterior and posterior portion. The anterior fibers are vertical; the posterior fibers are somewhat horizontal. The muscle inserts onto the coronoid process of the mandible and may also insert in the mandible distal to the mandibular third molar. Elevation of the mandible is accomplished when the entire muscle contracts. The mandible is retruded if any of the posterior fibers contract. It can be palpated above the zygomatic arch.

Masseter

This powerful muscle has a superficial and deep origin (Figures 18-1 and 18-2). The superficial fibers begin on the anterior two-thirds of the inferior border of the zygomatic arch. The deep fibers start from the posterior one-third of the zygomatic arch. The insertion of the deeper fibers is at the outside surface of the mandible and coronoid process of the mandible. The superficial fibers insert in the outer surface of the angle of the mandible. Contraction of this muscle causes the mandible to elevate. It is easily observed when the jaws are clenched.

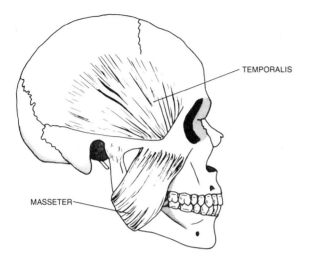

Figure 18-1 Muscles of mastication: masseter and temporalis

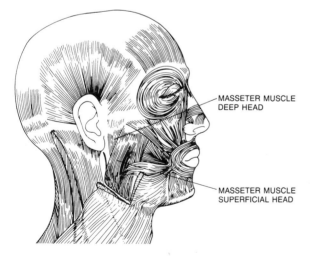

Figure 18-2 Masseter muscle, showing deep and superficial heads

Medial Pterygoid

This muscle also has a superficial and deep origin. The superficial fibers begin at the maxillary tuberosity, while the deep fibers arise from the medial side of the lateral pterygoid plate (Figures 18-3 and 18-4). The muscle inserts on the medial surface of the angle of the mandible. Its function is to elevate the mandible.

Lateral Pterygoid

The smaller, superior head starts from the infratemporal surface of the sphenoid bone and inserts into the articular disc of the temporomandibular joint (Figures 18-3 and 18-4). The larger, inferior head arises from the lateral surface of the lateral pterygoid plate and inserts in the pterygoid fovea of the mandible. Remember the origin of the medial pterygoid is the medial surface of the lateral pterygoid plate. If both pterygoid muscles contract, the jaw protrudes. If only one lateral pterygoid muscle contracts, there is a lateral shift of the mandible to the opposite side.

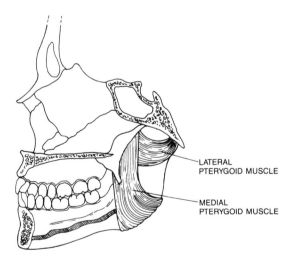

Figure 18-3 Medial and lateral pterygoid muscles, medial aspect

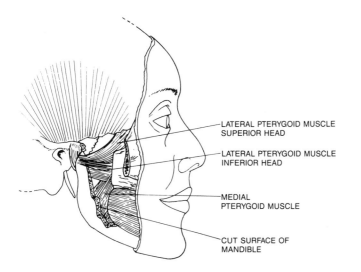

Figure 18-4 Pterygoid muscles, lateral aspect (coronoid process and anterior half of ramus or mandible removed)

SUPRAHYOID MUSCLES

These muscles are located above the hyoid bone. They are found between the mandible and the hyoid bone and function to lower the mandible or raise the hyoid bone.

Digastric

This slinglike muscle has fibers at either end and is connected in the center by an intermediate tendon or sling (Figures 18-5, 18-6, and 18-7). The anterior belly begins on the digastric fossa of the mandible (inferior surface of the mandible at the midline) and inserts into the intermediate tendon. The posterior belly starts from the intermediate tendon and inserts on the digastric notch (medial to the mastoid process). The anterior belly is innervated by the mandibular branch of the trigeminal nerve (V_3). The facial nerve (VII)* supplies the posterior belly.

*Refer to Chapter 19 for nerve designations.

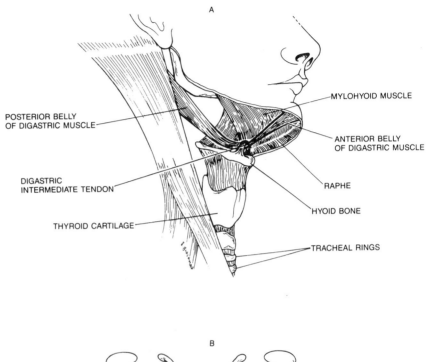

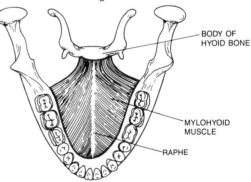

Figure 18-5 Mylohyoid muscle

Mylohyoid

This muscle creates the floor of the mouth (Figures 18-5, 18-6, and 18-7). It begins on the mylohyoid line of the mandible and inserts into a raphe at its midline. It is innervated by the mandibular branch of the trigeminal nerve.

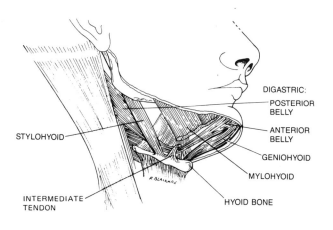

DIGASTRIC:
- POSTERIOR BELLY
- ANTERIOR BELLY

STYLOHYOID

GENIOHYOID

MYLOHYOID

INTERMEDIATE TENDON

HYOID BONE

Figure 18-6 Suprahyoid muscles

Geniohyoid

This muscle arises from the genial tubercles of the mandible and inserts on the hyoid bone (Figures 18-6 and 18-9). It is innervated by the hypoglossal nerve (XII), and is located above the mylohyoid muscle.

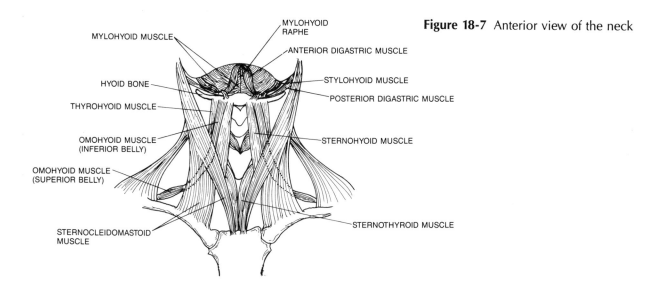

MYLOHYOID MUSCLE

HYOID BONE

THYROHYOID MUSCLE

OMOHYOID MUSCLE (INFERIOR BELLY)

OMOHYOID MUSCLE (SUPERIOR BELLY)

STERNOCLEIDOMASTOID MUSCLE

MYLOHYOID RAPHE

ANTERIOR DIGASTRIC MUSCLE

STYLOHYOID MUSCLE

POSTERIOR DIGASTRIC MUSCLE

STERNOHYOID MUSCLE

STERNOTHYROID MUSCLE

Figure 18-7 Anterior view of the neck

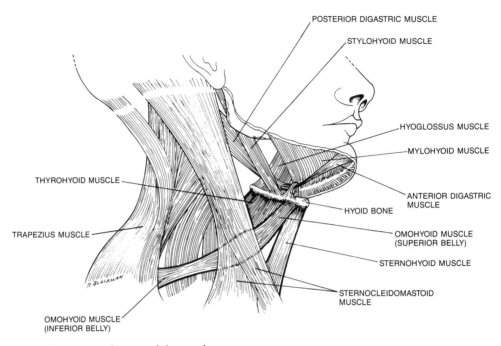

Figure 18-8 Lateral view of the neck

Stylohyoid

The origin of this muscle is the styloid process, while its insertion is the hyoid bone. It lies near the posterior belly of the digastric (Figures 18-6 through 18-9). It is innervated by the same branch of the facial nerve which supplies the posterior belly of the digastric.

INFRAHYOID MUSCLES

These muscles are located below the hyoid bone, in front of the neck. They function to depress the hyoid or fix it in place so the suprahyoid can work. They are innervated by the first, second, and third cervical nerves.

Omohyoid

This muscle has two bellies that are joined by an intermediate tendon (Figures 18-7 and 18-8). The inferior belly comes from the scapula and ends on the

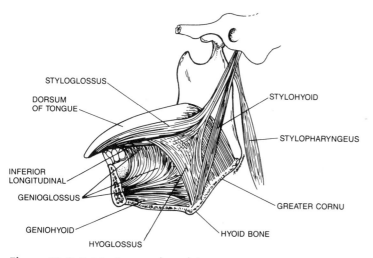

STYLOGLOSSUS

DORSUM
OF TONGUE

STYLOHYOID

STYLOPHARYNGEUS

INFERIOR
LONGITUDINAL

GENIOGLOSSUS

GREATER CORNU

GENIOHYOID

HYOID BONE

HYOGLOSSUS

Figure 18-9 Extrinsic muscles of the tongue

intermediate tendon, while the superior belly originates on the intermediate tendon and inserts on the hyoid bone.

Sternohyoid

The origin of this muscle is the sternum and its insertion is the hyoid bone (Figures 18-7 and 18-8).

Sternothyroid

This muscle arises from the sternum and inserts on the thyroid cartilage (Figure 18-7). It is located below the sternohyoid.

Thyrohyoid

The thyrohyoid originates on the thyroid cartilage and inserts on the hyoid bone (Figure 18-8).

MUSCLES OF THE TONGUE

The muscles of the tongue are divided into two groups, intrinsic and extrinsic. These muscles help the tongue to change its shape and position. Tongue muscles are innervated by the hypoglossal nerve (XII).

Intrinsic Muscles

These muscles lie in and are contained entirely within the tongue. They are responsible for changes in the shape of the tongue and are named for the direction in which they run.

Superior Longitudinal

This muscle runs the length of the tongue from anterior to posterior. It is located near the top of the tongue, and functions to widen the tongue and turn the tip up.

Inferior Longitudinal

This muscle also runs the length of the tongue from anterior to posterior; however, it lies near the bottom of the tongue (Figure 18-9). It also widens the tongue, but turns the tip down.

Transverse

This muscle is found on the lateral edges of the tongue. Its function is to make the tongue narrow.

Vertical

This muscle runs from the upper surface to the lower surface of the tongue. It aids in widening the tongue tip.

Extrinsic Muscles

These muscles originate from close structures and insert on or intermingle with intrinsic muscles. They aid in positioning the tongue.

Genioglossus

The origin of this muscle is the genial tubercles and its insertion is on the tongue and hyoid bone (Figure 18-9). Anterior fibers retract the tongue and posterior fibers push it forward. This muscle does a majority of work for the tongue.

Hyoglossus

This muscle originates on the hyoid bone and inserts on the side of the tongue. It depresses the tongue and draws the sides down.

Styloglossus

This muscle is from the styloid process and has two insertions on the tongue. One head intermingles with the inferior longitudinal and the other joins with the hyoglossus. The styloglossus draws the tongue up and backward.

Palatoglossus

This muscle forms the anterior tonsillar arch (in front of the tonsils). Its origin is the underside of the soft palate and its insertion is the posterior side of the tongue. It is innervated by the pharyngeal plexus, a group of branches from the glossopharyngeal (IX), vagus (X) and spinal accessory (XI) nerves. Its contraction pulls the sides of the tongue faucial up and back, and the soft palate down. It also constricts the pillars.

MUSCLES OF FACIAL EXPRESSION

Contraction of these muscles results in a wide variety of facial expressions. The facial nerve (VII) provides innervation to these muscles. These muscles are symmetrical and work in groups.

Muscles of the Scalp

The *occipitofrontalis (epicranius)* is made up of two groups, the *frontalis* and *occipitalis* (Figure 18-10). This muscle pulls the scalp forward and backward and raises the eyebrows.

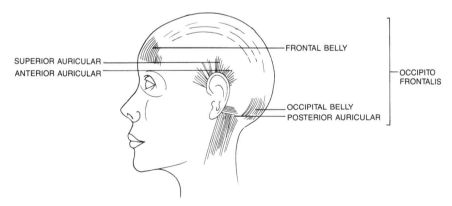

Figure 18-10 Three groups of auricular muscles around the ear

Muscles of the Ears

There are three groups of ear muscles: *anterior auricular, posterior auricular,* and *superior auricular* (Figure 18-10). They are respectively located in front of, behind, and above the ear. These muscles may draw the ear forward and backward or elevate the ear.

Orbicularis Oculi

This muscle encircles the eye. It is divided into an orbital and palpebral (eyelid) section, and functions to close the eyes.

Procerus

This muscle runs from the bridge of the nose to the eyebrow (Figure 18-11). It pulls the eyebrows downward.

Figure 18-11 Muscles of eye and nose

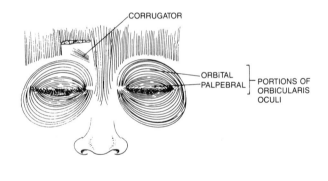

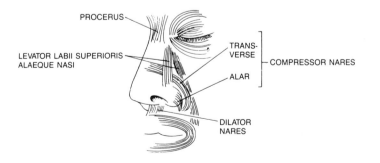

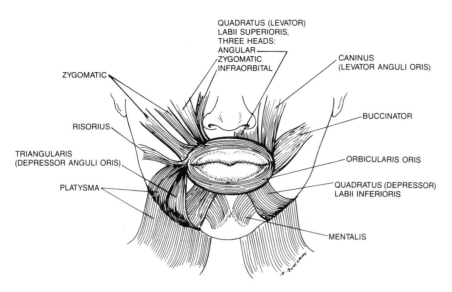

Figure 18-12 Muscles of expression in lower face

Corrugator

The *corrugator* runs along the eyebrow and inserts on the medial end of the eyebrow (Figure 18-11). It pulls the eyebrow down and in.

Muscles of the Nose

The *nasalis* is divided into two parts: the *compressor nares* and the *dilator nares* (Figure 18-11). The *dilator nares* cause flaring of the nostrils. The *compressor nares* close the nostrils.

Muscles of the Mouth

Orbicularis oris. This muscle has no skeletal attachment. It encircles the mouth and composes the lips (Figure 18-12). Its function is to close the lips or protrude them. Its fibers interlace with other perioral muscles.

Levator Labii Superioris Alaeque Nasi. This tiny muscle inserts on the ala of the nose and runs to the upper lip (Figure 18-13). It raises the upper lip.

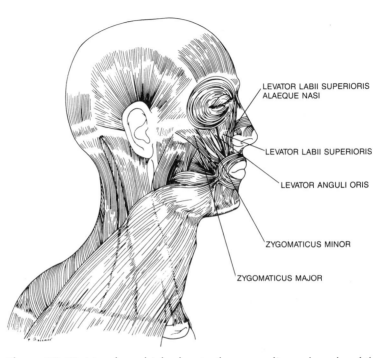

LEVATOR LABII SUPERIORIS
ALAEQUE NASI

LEVATOR LABII SUPERIORIS

LEVATOR ANGULI ORIS

ZYGOMATICUS MINOR

ZYGOMATICUS MAJOR

Figure 18-13 Muscles which elevate the upper lip and angle of the mouth

Levator Labii Superioris or *Quadratus Labii Superioris.* This muscle runs above the mouth and has three heads:

1. *angular* — near the nose
2. *infraorbital* — lower edge of orbit
3. *zygomatic* — zygomatic bone

All heads insert onto the upper lip and these muscles help elevate the upper lip (Figure 18-13).

Zygomatic. Its origin is the zygomatic bone and it inserts into the corner of the mouth or the *modiolus,* an area of intertwining muscles. It elevates the angle of the mouth up and laterally. It may be divided into zygomatic major and minor muscles (Figures 18-12 and 18-13).

Levator Anguli Oris or *Caninus.* Its origin is the canine fossa, a depression near the canine roots below the infraorbital foramen. It inserts into the *modiolus* and aids in elevating the corner of the mouth (Figures 18-12, 18-13, and 18-14).

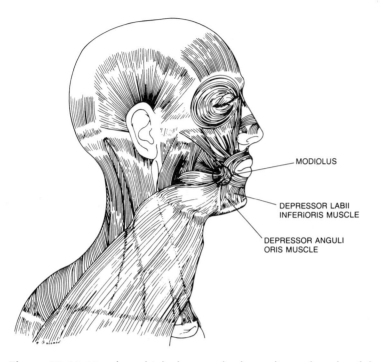

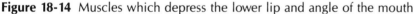

Figure 18-14 Muscles which depress the lower lip and angle of the mouth

Buccinator. This muscle forms the cheek (Figure 18-15). It originates from the alveolar process of the mandible, maxilla, and the pterygomandibular raphe, a fibrous band that runs from the pterygoid hamulus to the mylohyoid line. It blends with the orbicularis oris at the modiolus. The *buccinator* holds the cheek against the teeth and keeps food on the occlusal surfaces during mastication.

Risorius. It originates on the anterior border of the masseter muscle and inserts into the modiolus (Figure 18-12). It pulls the angle of the mouth laterally and aids in smiling.

Depressor Anguli Oris or *Triangularis.* This muscle arises from the external oblique line of the mandible and inserts into the modiolus (Figure 18-12). It pulls the corner of the mouth downward and inward.

Depressor Labii Inferioris or *Quadratus Labii Inferioris.* This muscle also arises from the external oblique line; however, it inserts into the skin of the lower lip (Figures 18-12 and 18-14). It functions to pull the lower lip down and laterally.

Mentalis. This is the only muscle whose fibers run away from the lips (Figure 18-12). Its origin is a fossa or depression beneath the mandibular anterior teeth and it inserts into the skin of the chin. It can raise the skin of the chin and protrude the lower lip.

MUSCLES OF THE NECK

Platysma

The platysma is a thin sheet of muscle located just below the skin of the neck (Figures 18-15 and 18-16). Its origin is the clavicle and shoulder; it travels upward to insert on the lower border of the mandible as well as the skin and muscle of the lower face and mouth. Contraction of this muscle wrinkles the skin of the chin and neck and draws the outer part of the lower lip down and back. It is innervated by the facial nerve (VII).

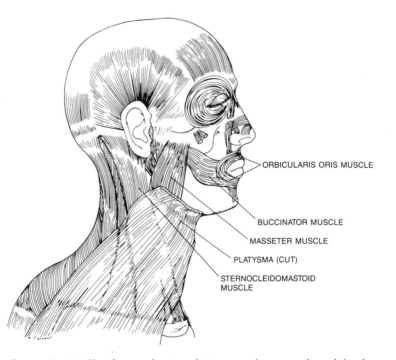

ORBICULARIS ORIS MUSCLE

BUCCINATOR MUSCLE

MASSETER MUSCLE

PLATYSMA (CUT)

STERNOCLEIDOMASTOID MUSCLE

Figure 18-15 Cheek muscles in relation to other muscles of the face and neck

Trapezius

This is a large muscle covering the back of the neck, shoulder, and clavicle (Figures 18-8 and 18-16). It originates from the external occipital protuberance and it inserts into the clavicle and shoulder. This muscle moves the head backward and laterally. The spinal accessory nerve (XI) provides innervation to this muscle.

Sternocleidomastoid

This prominent muscle arises by two heads, from the top of the sternum and clavicle (Figures 18-7, 18-8, 18-15, and 18-16). The two heads blend together and insert on the mastoid process and the superior nunchal line of the occipital bone. This muscle turns the chin upward to the opposite side when the head is turned laterally. Innervation is provided by the spinal accessory nerve (XI).

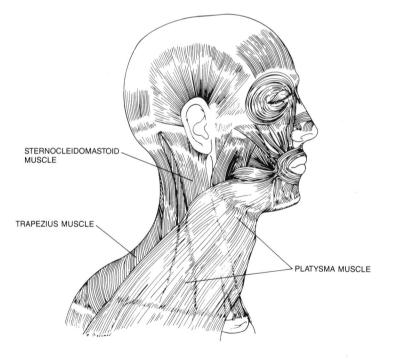

STERNOCLEIDOMASTOID
MUSCLE

TRAPEZIUS MUSCLE

PLATYSMA MUSCLE

Figure 18-16 Platysma muscle, lateral aspect

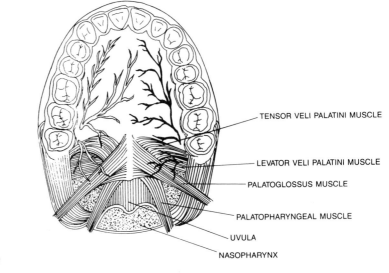

TENSOR VELI PALATINI MUSCLE

LEVATOR VELI PALATINI MUSCLE

PALATOGLOSSUS MUSCLE

PALATOPHARYNGEAL MUSCLE

UVULA

NASOPHARYNX

Figure 18-17 Muscles of the soft palate

MUSCLES OF THE SOFT PALATE

These muscles raise the soft palate during *deglutition* or swallowing.

Palatoglossus or Palatoglossal

This muscle was discussed previously under Extrinsic Tongue Muscles. It is associated with both the tongue and the soft palate (Figures 18-17 and 18-18). It forms the anterior tonsillar pillar.

Palatopharyngeal

This muscle forms the posterior tonsillar pillar (Figures 18-17, 18-18, and 18-19). Contraction of this muscle causes the pharynx to elevate. It is innervated by the pharyngeal plexus.

Uvula

This small mass of tissue hangs down in the throat from the soft palate (Figures 18-17 and 18-19). Upon contraction, the *uvula* will shorten. Innervation is through the pharyngeal plexus.

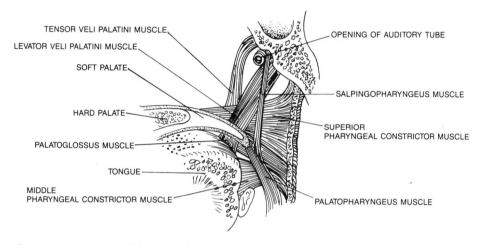

Figure 18-18 View of the lateral throat wall looking from the midline

Levator Veli Palatini

This muscle originates from the petrous portion of the temporal bone, and it inserts in the soft palate (Figures 18-17, 18-18, and 18-19). It pulls the soft palate upward and back, and is innervated by the pharyngeal plexus.

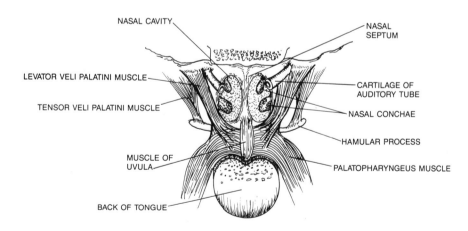

Figure 18-19 Posterior view of the muscles of the soft palate

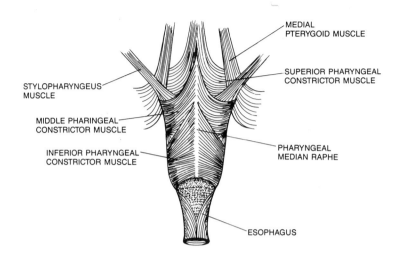

Figure 18-20 Posterior view of the pharyngeal wall

Tensor Veli Palatini

This muscle arises from the medial pterygoid plate and auditory tube (Figures 18-17, 18-18, and 18-19). It turns upward, curves around the pterygoid hamulus, and then inserts into the soft palate. It tenses (hence the name) the soft palate by pulling on the lateral sides. It is innervated by the mandibular branch of the trigeminal nerve (V_3).

MUSCLES OF THE PHARYNX

The pharynx is a muscular tube. It is made up of three constrictor muscles and three smaller muscles. All of the muscles function in deglutition or swallowing. All constrictors are innervated by the pharyngeal plexus.

Superior Constrictor

The origin of this muscle is the pterygoid hamulus, medial pterygoid plate, pterygomandibular raphe, and the mylohyoid line (Figures 18-18 and 18-20). All three constrictors insert and unite on the *median raphe*.

Middle Constrictor

The greater and lesser horns of the hyoid bone and the stylohyoid ligament are the origins for this muscle (Figures 18-18 and 18-20). It unites with the superior constrictor at the median raphe.

Inferior Constrictor

This muscle arises from the thyroid cartilage of the larynx (Figure 18-20). Its fibers join at the median raphe. Fibers of all three constrictors overlap each other.

Palatopharyngeal

Previously, this muscle was discussed as a muscle of the soft palate. Its function is to elevate the pharynx, so it is also listed here under muscles of the pharynx.

Elevators and Dilators of the Pharynx

Salpingopharyngeal. The origin of this muscle is the auditory tube (Figure 18-18). Its fibers blend with the palatopharyngeal muscle. It helps to elevate the pharynx and it is innervated by the pharyngeal plexus.

Stylopharyngeal. This muscle arises from the styloid process and inserts on the thyroid cartilage (Figure 18-20). It helps to elevate and dilate the pharynx. Innervation is supplied by the glossopharyngeal nerve (IX).

Deglutition

Swallowing is divided into three stages: *oral*, *pharyngeal*, and *esophageal*.

Oral Stage. During the *oral stage* of swallowing, the bolus, a ball of chewed food mixed with saliva, is centered on the tongue. The tongue is then raised up and back and a seal is made between the hard palate and the tongue. The sides of the tongue seal against the teeth and the mucosa of the hard palate. The bolus is moved backward by the intrinsic and extrinsic muscles of the tongue, as well as the suprahyoid muscles. The muscles of mastication hold the teeth together. The bolus is now positioned onto the posterior tongue. The upward and backward movement of the tongue causes the muscles of the soft palate to elevate the soft palate.

Pharyngeal Stage. The fauces are narrowed by the palatoglossal muscle. The soft palate contacts the posterior pharyngeal wall. The stylopharyngeal and salpingopharyngeal muscles elevate and dilate the pharynx to make room for the bolus that has just entered the pharynx. The superior, middle, and inferior constrictors squeeze the pharynx, propelling the bolus into the lower end of the pharynx.

The thyroid cartilage of the larynx is raised and brought forward by the thyrohyoid muscle and other muscles. The epiglottis protects the larynx from the bolus. The food is then propelled into the upper part of the esophagus.

Esophageal Stage. The bolus is propelled by peristaltic contractions into the stomach.

SUMMARY

The muscles of the head and neck are divided into eight groups: (1) the *muscles of mastication*, including the temporalis, masseter, and medial and lateral pterygoid, which cause the movement of the mandible; (2) the *suprahyoid muscles*, including the digastric, mylohyoid, geniohyoid, and stylohyoid, which cause movement of the lower mandible and raise the hyoid bone; (3) *infrahyoid muscles*, including omohyoid, sternohyoid, sternothyroid, and thyrohyoid, which depress the hyoid bone or hold it in place so the suprahyoids can work; (4) the *muscles of the tongue*, including the various intrinsic muscles, which change the shape of the tongue, and the various extrinsic muscles, which position the tongue; (5) the *muscles of facial expression*, including the various muscles of the scalp, ear, eye, nose, and neck, which control facial expression; (6) the *muscles of the neck*, including the platysma, trapezius, and sternocleidomastoid, which control the movement of the head, chin, neck, and lips; (7) the *muscles of the soft palate*, including the palatoglossal, palatopharyngeal, uvula, and the levator and tensor veli palatini, which raise the soft palate during swallowing; (8) the *muscles of the pharynx*, including the superior, middle, and inferior constrictors, palatopharyngeal, salpingo pharyngeal, and stylopharyngeal, which control swallowing, allowing the elevation and dilation of the pharynx.

WORKSHEET

A. Define the following terms.

origin

insertion

modiolus

deglutition

B. Complete the chart on the Muscles of Mastication.

MUSCLE	ORIGIN	INSERTION	FUNCTION
Masseter			
Temporalis			
Lateral Pterygoid			
Medial Pterygoid			

C. List the steps that occur during each phase of swallowing.

D. Complete the following figures.

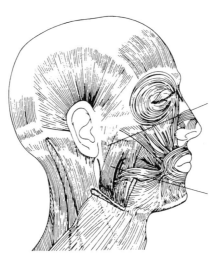

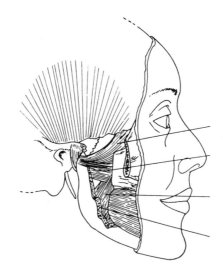

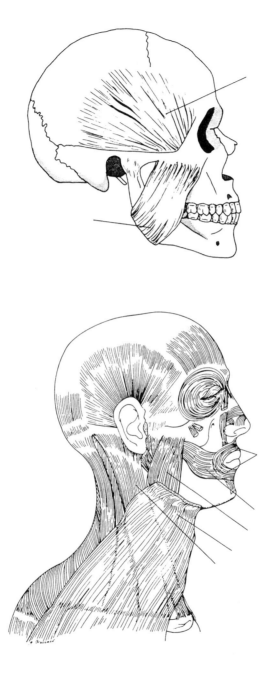

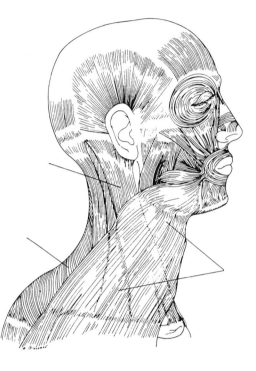

E. Answer the following questions.

1. Name the suprahyoid and infrahyoid muscles.

2. What nerve innervates the muscles of mastication?

3. What nerve innervates the muscles of facial expression?

4. The contraction of what muscle of mastication causes the mandible to swing to the side?

5. What muscle forms the cheek?

19

Nerves of the Head and Neck

Objectives

- List the names and numbers of the cranial nerves.
- Describe the following terms: neuron, dendrite, axon, efferent, afferent, somatic, and visceral.
- Describe the central, peripheral, and autonomic nervous systems.
- Differentiate between sympathetic and parasympathetic nerve supply.
- Describe the trigeminal, facial, glossopharyngeal, and hypoglossal nerves according to the following: nerve supply (sensory, motor or both), structures supplied, teeth supplied, and exit site.
- Describe nerve supply to each maxillary and mandibular tooth.
- Complete the worksheet at the end of the chapter.

INTRODUCTION

Our nervous system has two parts: the *central nervous system* (CNS) and the *peripheral nervous system* (PNS). The central nervous system is further classified into: the *brain*, which is housed in the cranium, and the *spinal cord*, which is contained within the vertebral column. The peripheral nervous system is made up of the nerves that travel away from the central nervous system. There are 12 pairs of *cranial* nerves and 31 pairs of *spinal nerves* in the peripheral nervous system. Through the peripheral nervous system, all parts of the body are connected to the central nervous system.

A nerve cell is also known as a *neuron*. A neuron has three parts (Figure 19-1):

1. Cell body

2. Dendrite — a process that conducts impulses toward the cell body. A neuron may have one or many dendrites.

3. Axon — a process that carries impulses away from the cell body. A neuron has only one axon.

Nerves that carry impulses or messages toward the brain are known as *sensory* or *afferent.* Those nerves that carry impulses away from the brain are

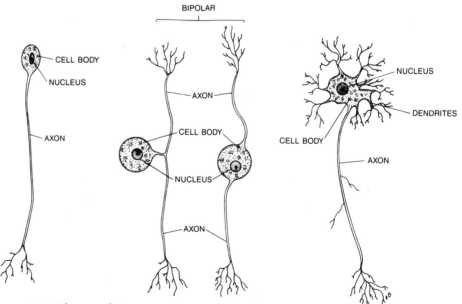

Figure 19-1 Shapes of Neurons

termed *motor* or *efferent. Somatic* nerves supply muscles, while *visceral* nerves provide innervation to the internal organs (viscera).

The *autonomic nervous system* controls those functions over which we have no control, such as heart rate and respiratory rate. This nervous system is divided into two parts: *sympathetic* and *parasympathetic.*

Usually each organ has sympathetic and parasympathetic nerves supplying it. These systems tend to produce opposite actions.

The sympathetic system functions in response to emergencies. Sympathetic nerves increase respiration, heart rate, and blood flow to muscles. They decrease salivary flow and blood supply to the digestive tract in order that additional blood can be supplied to other muscles. This is often referred to as the "fight or flight" reaction.

The parasympathetic system slows down the heart and respiration; these nerves increase blood to the digestive system and salivary glands.

THE CRANIAL NERVES

As mentioned before, there are twelve sets of (or "paired") cranial nerves. They provide innervation to the right and left sides of the body, and are designated by a Roman numeral. They may be entirely sensory, entirely motor, or a combination of both sensory and motor (mixed). This text concentrates on four cranial nerves that are important for dental auxiliaries: the trigeminal (V), facial (VII), glossopharyngeal (IX), and hypoglossal (XII). The remaining cranial nerves appear in Table 19-1.

THE TRIGEMINAL NERVE (V) (Mixed)

This is the largest cranial nerve and the most important to dental auxiliaries because it provides sensory innervation from the face, scalp, teeth, nose, and mouth. It also distributes motor innervation to the muscles of mastication and provides parasympathetic supply to the salivary and lacrimal glands. Sensory cells are located in the semilunar (gasserian) ganglion found in the petrous portion of the temporal bone. The motor root originates in the pons and joins the mandibular division. The trigeminal nerve has three divisions or branches (Figure 19-2):

1. Ophthalmic nerve (V_1) — entirely afferent
2. Maxillary nerve (V_2) — entirely afferent
3. Mandibular nerve (V_3) — mixed, both afferent and efferent.

CRANIAL NERVE	SENSORY (S) MOTOR (M) BOTH (B)	FUNCTION	EXIT SITE
Olfactory I	S	Sense of smell	Cribiform plate
Optic II	S	Sight	Optic foramen (canal)
Oculomotor III	M	Motor to extrinsic eye muscles (superior and inferior rectus muscles and inferior oblique)	Superior orbital fissure
Trochlear IV	M	Motor to superior oblique eye muscle	Superior orbital fissure
Abducent VI	M	Motor to lateral rectus eye muscle	Superior orbital fissure
Acoustic VII	S	Hearing and balance	Internal acoustic (auditory) meatus
Vagus X	B	Longest cranial nerve. Sensory innervation to ear, pharynx, larynx, bronchi, lungs, heart, esophagus, stomach, intestines, and kidney. Parasympathetic control of heart rate. Contributes to pharyngeal plexus.	Jugular foramen
(Spinal) Accessory XI	M	Has a cranial and spinal part. Associated with vagus (X) nerve. Contributes to pharyngeal plexus. Motor to trapezius and sternocleidomastoid muscles.	Jugular foramen

Table 19-1. Other Cranial Nerves

The Ophthalmic Nerve

This nerve enters the eye through the *superior orbital fissure* and provides sensory innervation to the eye, nose, lacrimal gland, and skin of the eyelids, forehead, and nose. There are no branches to the oral cavity. It has three branches:

> 1. *Lacrimal nerve* — innervates the lacrimal glands for tear production and supplies the skin of the upper eyelid

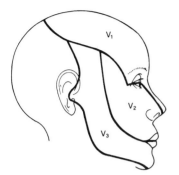

Figure 19-2 Area of distribution of the three divisions of the trigeminal nerve

2. *Frontal nerve* —.passes above the eye dividing into the *supraorbital* and *supratrochlear* nerves. The supraorbital branch supplies the skin of the forehead, scalp, and upper eyelid. The supratrochlear branch supplies the skin of the forehead and upper eyelid (Figure 19-3).

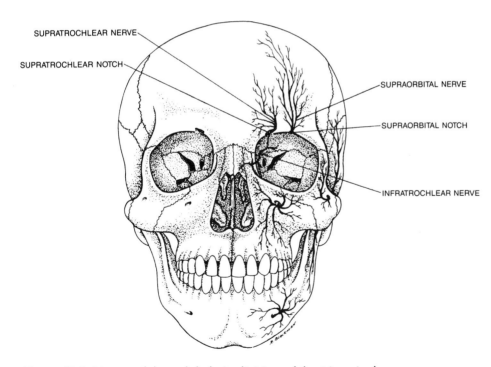

Figure 19-3 Nerves of the ophthalmic division of the trigeminal nerve

3. *Nasociliary nerve* — runs within the orbit, passes through the ethmoid bone, and reenters the cranium at the cribiform plate of the ethmoid bone. It then passes down into the nose and supplies the inside of the nose and skin on the side of the nose.

The Maxillary Nerve

The second division of the trigeminal nerve exits the skull through the *foramen rotundum* and passes into the pterygopalatine fossa. In this fossa, the maxillary nerve divides into four branches: *zygomatic, infraorbital, posterior superior alveolar* (PSA), and *pterygopalatine.*

The Zygomatic Nerve. This nerve enters the eye through the *inferior orbital fissure.* It has two branches (Figure 19-4):

1. *Zygomaticotemporal* — supplies the skin and side of the forehead
2. *Zygomaticofacial* — supplies skin of the cheek

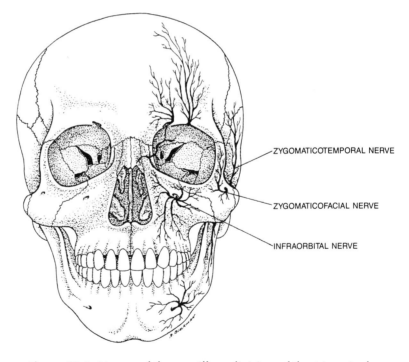

ZYGOMATICOTEMPORAL NERVE

ZYGOMATICOFACIAL NERVE

INFRAORBITAL NERVE

Figure 19-4 Nerves of the maxillary division of the trigeminal nerve

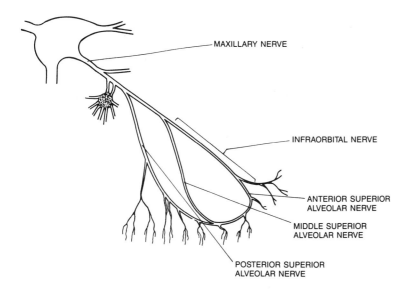

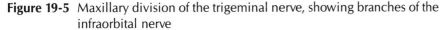

Figure 19-5 Maxillary division of the trigeminal nerve, showing branches of the infraorbital nerve

The Infraorbital Nerve. This nerve emerges onto the face through the *infraorbital foramen* on the maxilla, but before this nerve exits through the infraorbital foramen it gives off two descending branches (Figures 19-5 and 19-6).

1. *The Middle Superior Alveolar* (MSA) nerve provides innervation to the mesio-buccal root of the maxillary first molar, the maxillary first and second premolars, the adjacent gingiva, and the maxillary sinus. The middle superior alveolar nerve is not always present. If it is not present, innervation to that area is provided by the anterior and posterior superior alveolar nerves (Figures 19-5 and 19-6).

2. *The Anterior Superior Alveolar* (ASA) nerve supplies the maxillary incisor and canine teeth and associated labial gingiva. It also innervates the maxillary sinus (Figures 19-5 and 19-6).

After the infraorbital nerve emerges onto the face through the infraorbital foramen, it divides into three terminal branches:

1. *Palpebral* — supplies the skin of the lower eyelid
2. *External nasal* — innervates the skin and mucosa of the side of the nose
3. *Superior labial* — supplies skin and mucosa of the upper lid and labial mucosa (Figure 19-6)

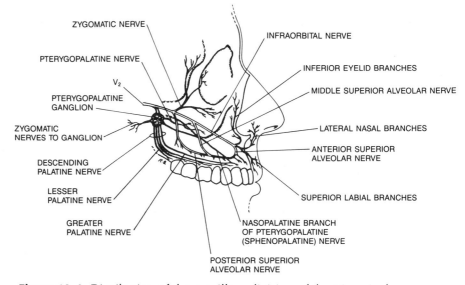

Figure 19-6 Distribution of the maxillary division of the trigeminal nerve

Posterior Superior Alveolar (PSA) Nerve. Before the infraorbital nerve enters the intraorbital groove, it gives off the posterior superior alveolar nerve (Figures 19-5 and 19-6). This nerve crosses the maxillary tuberosity and supplies the maxillary molar teeth, with the exception of the mesiobuccal root of the maxillary first molar which is innervated by the middle superior alveolar nerve (MSA). The adjacent buccal gingiva and maxillary sinus are also supplied by the posterior superior alveolar nerves.

Pterygopalatine Nerves. Five branches of the maxillary nerve are given off in the pterygopalatine fossa (Figure 19-6).

1. *Pharyngeal* — supplies the pharynx and pharyngeal mucosa
2. *Greater palatine* — enters the greater palatine foramen (palatine bone) to supply the mucosa of the hard palate and lingual gingiva of the maxillary molars, premolars, and canine teeth
3. *Lesser palatine* — enters the lesser palatine foramen to supply the mucosa of the soft palate and tonsils
4. *Nasopalatine* — passes through the nasopalatine (incisive) foramen of the maxilla to supply the lingual gingiva of the maxillary incisor teeth
5. *Posterior superior lateral nasal* — supplies the middle and superior nasal conchae and the superior nasal septum

The Mandibular Nerve

The mandibular nerve is the largest division of the trigeminal nerve and exits the skull through the *foramen ovale* in the sphenoid bone. It is both afferent and efferent.

After the foramen ovale, the sensory and motor roots of the mandibular nerve unite in a short trunk. The sensory branch gives off the *meningeal nerve* which passes through the foramen spinosum to supply the meninges. The motor branch distributes nerves to the following muscles: *medial pterygoid, tensor tympani,* and *tensor veli palatini.* The mandibular nerve then branches into anterior and posterior divisions.

The Anterior Division. This division has only one sensory branch; the remaining nerves are all motor to the muscles of mastication (Figure 19-7).

Motor

- *Masseteric nerve* — supplies masseter muscle
- *Anterior and posterior deep temporal nerves* — supply the temporalis muscle
- *Lateral pterygoid nerve* — supplies the lateral pterygoid muscle

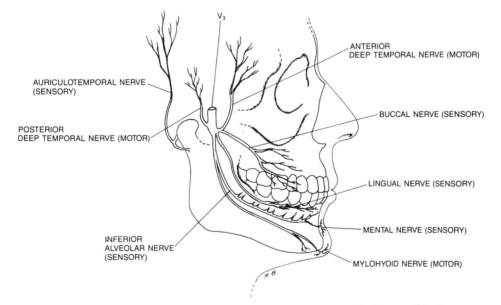

Figure 19-7 Inferior alveolar nerve enters the mandible through the mandibular foramen; mental nerve branches off it in the premolar region.

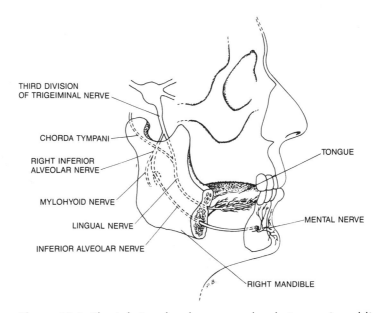

THIRD DIVISION
OF TRIGEIMINAL NERVE

CHORDA TYMPANI

RIGHT INFERIOR
ALVEOLAR NERVE

MYLOHYOID NERVE

LINGUAL NERVE

INFERIOR ALVEOLAR NERVE

TONGUE

MENTAL NERVE

RIGHT MANDIBLE

Figure 19-8 The inferior alveolar nerve, chorda tympani, and lingual nerve

Sensory

The *buccal (long buccal) nerve* is the only sensory nerve in the anterior division. It crosses between the two heads of the lateral pterygoid muscle and emerges through the buccinator muscle. It innervates the buccal gingiva of the mandibular molars, the mucosa of the cheek, and the skin of the cheek.

The Posterior Division. This division has only one motor branch; the remaining branches are all sensory.

The *auriculotemporal nerve* supplies the skin of the temporal region in front of the ear, external acoustic (auditory) meatus, and the temporomandibular joint (Figure 19-7). After giving off the auriculotemporal nerve, the mandibular nerve divides into two terminal branches.

The *lingual nerve* runs between the medial pterygoid muscle and the mandible. It is joined by the *chorda tympani*, a branch of the facial nerve (VII). Together the lingual and chorda tympani nerves enter the posterior aspect of the mouth and run forward. The *chorda tympani* supplies taste sensation to the anterior two-thirds of the tongue. The lingual nerve enters the floor of the mouth and ventral surface of the tongue. It supplies afferent innervation to the tongue, floor of the mouth, and lingual gingiva of the entire mandibular arch. Remember the chorda tympani provides taste to the anterior two-thirds of the tongue (Figures 19-6, 19-8, and 19-9).

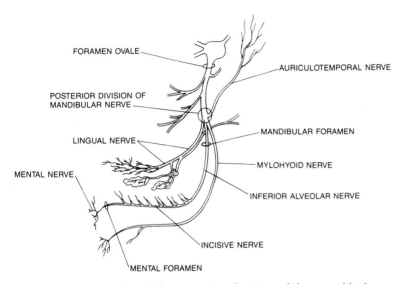

Figure 19-9 Branches of the posterior division of the mandibular nerve

Inferior Alveolar Nerve. This nerve runs parallel with the lingual nerve. It then enters the mandible through the mandibular foramen and continues in the mandibular canal. Before it enters the mandibular foramen, it gives off the *mylohyoid nerve,* the only motor branch in the posterior division. It supplies efferent sensation to the mylohyoid muscle and the anterior belly of the digastric muscle. After giving off the mylohyoid nerve, the inferior alveolar nerve is entirely sensory.

Within the mandibular canal, the inferior alveolar nerve gives off branches to the mandibular molars and premolars. At the *mental foramen,* it divides into the:

- *Mental nerve,* which supplies the chin and lower lip (Figures 19-7 and 19-9)
- *Incisive nerve,* which supplies the mandibular anterior teeth and labial gingiva (Figures 19-7 and 19-9).

THE FACIAL NERVE (VII)

The facial nerve is both afferent and efferent. It provides motor innervation to all the muscles of facial expression, posterior belly of the digastric muscle, stylohyoid, and stapedius muscle of the middle ear. It also provides taste sensation to the anterior two-thirds of the tongue and sensory innervation to the nose and salivary glands.

This nerve enters the internal acoustic meatus and travels through the temporal bone. The facial nerve encounters its sensory ganglion, the *geniculate ganglion*, in the temporal bone. While in the temporal bone, the facial nerve gives off the following branches:

- *Greater petrosal nerve* — supplies efferent innervation to glands of the nose and mouth and the lacrimal gland
- *Nerve to the stapedius muscle* — supplies the stapedius muscle of the inner ear
- *Chorda tympani nerve* — joins with the lingual nerve and carries taste fibers to the anterior two-thirds of the tongue (Figure 19-8)

The facial nerve then exits the skull through the stylomastoid foramen and gives off the following branches:

- *Posterior auricular nerve* — supplies the posterior auricular and occipital muscles
- *Digastric nerve* — provides innervation to the posterior belly of the digastric muscle
- *Stylohyoid nerve* — innervates the stylohyoid muscle

The facial nerve then enters the *parotid gland*. It bifurcates into two divisions, a superior *temporofacial* and an inferior *cervicofacial* (Figure 19-10). The temporofacial division gives rise to:

- *Temporal branches* — supply the anterior and superior auricular muscles, frontal muscle, corrugator muscle of the eyebrow, and the orbicularis oculi
- *Zygomatic branches* — also provide innervation to the orbicularis oculi
- *Buccal branches* — supply procerus, zygomatic, quadratus labii superioris, nasalis, buccinator, orbicularis oris, and risorius muscles

The *cervicofacial trunk* gives rise to:

- *Mandibular branch* — provides innervation to the muscles of the lower lip and chin
- *Cervical branch* — supplies the platysma muscle

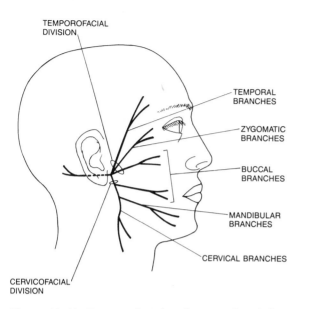

TEMPOROFACIAL
DIVISION

TEMPORAL
BRANCHES

ZYGOMATIC
BRANCHES

BUCCAL
BRANCHES

MANDIBULAR
BRANCHES

CERVICAL BRANCHES

CERVICOFACIAL
DIVISION

Figure 19-10 Temporofacial and cervicofacial divisions of the facial nerve

THE GLOSSOPHARYNGEAL NERVE (IX)

The glossopharyngeal nerve is both afferent and efferent, and it exits the skull through the jugular foramen. Its branches are distributed to the tongue and pharynx. The branches of the glossopharyngeal nerve include:

- *Tympanic nerve* — provides parasympathetic innervation to the parotid gland and sensory innervation to the middle ear
- *Carotid sinus nerve* — supplies afferent innervation to the carotid sinus for its blood pressure regulators
- *Stylopharyngeal nerve* — supplies motor innervation to the stylopharyngeal muscle
- *Pharyngeal branches* — join with the spinal accessory (XI) and vagus (X) nerves to create the *pharyngeal plexus*. This plexus supplies the muscle of the soft palate and pharynx, except for the stylopharyngeal supplied by (IX) and tensor veli palatini innervated by (V). It also innervates the mucosa of the soft palate, pharynx, and tonsils. The glossopharyngeal nerve also supplies the posterior one-third of the tongue with taste sensation.

THE HYPOGLOSSAL NERVE (XII)

This nerve is the motor supply of the tongue. It exits the skull through the hypoglossal canal and is entirely efferent. It enters the mouth to supply the geniohyoid muscle and intrinsic and extrinsic muscles of the tongue except the palatoglossal muscle which is innervated by the pharyngeal plexus. Damage to this nerve causes paralysis of the tongue. The tongue will deviate toward the affected side when protruded.

SUMMARY

The peripheral nervous system is made up of the nerves that travel *away from* the central nervous system; it *connects* all parts of the body with the central nervous system. There are twelve pairs of cranial nerves and thirty-one pairs of spinal nerves in the peripheral nervous system.

The cranial nerves provide innervation to the right and left side of the body, and they are usually designated by a Roman numeral. The major cranial nerves include (1) the *trigeminal nerve*, which innervates the face, scalp, teeth, nose, mouth, and muscles of mastication and includes three branches — the ophthalmic nerve, the maxillary nerve, and the mandibular nerve; (2) the *facial nerve*, which innervates the muscles of facial expression, the muscles of the middle ear, and provides sensory innervation to the tongue, nose, and salivary glands and divides into eight branches — greater petrosal, nerve to stapedius muscle, chorda tympani, posterior auricular, digastric, stylohyoid, temporofacial, and cervicofacial; (3) the *glossopharyngeal nerve*, which supplies the posterior third of the tongue with taste and includes four branches — the tympanic, carotid sinus, stylopharyngeal, and pharyngeal; (4) the *hypoglossal nerve*, which innervates the geniohyoid, and the intrinsic and extrinsic muscles of the tongue.

WORKSHEET

A. *Define the following terms.*
    sympathetic
    parasympathetic
    afferent
    efferent

B. Complete the following chart.

Nerve	Sensory (S) Motor (M) Both (B)	Function	Exit Site

Trigeminal
  Ophthalmic (V$_1$)
  Maxillary (V$_2$)
  Mandibular (V$_3$)			

Facial			
Glossopharyngeal			
Hypoglossal			

C. Trace a pain impulse from the foramen rotundum to the maxillary right first molar.

D. Complete the following figures.

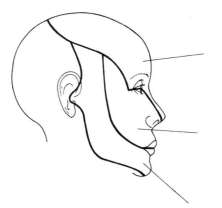

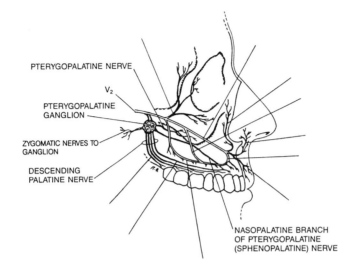

PTERYGOPALATINE NERVE

V₂

PTERYGOPALATINE
GANGLION

ZYGOMATIC NERVES TO
GANGLION

DESCENDING
PALATINE NERVE

NASOPALATINE BRANCH
OF PTERYGOPALATINE
(SPHENOPALATINE) NERVE

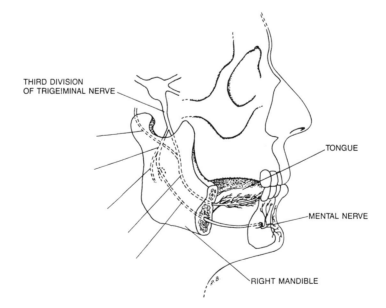

THIRD DIVISION
OF TRIGEIMINAL NERVE

TONGUE

MENTAL NERVE

RIGHT MANDIBLE

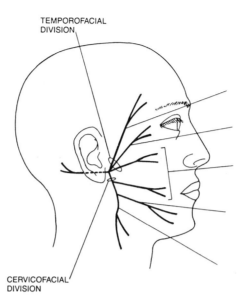

TEMPOROFACIAL DIVISION

CERVICOFACIAL DIVISION

E. Answer the following questions and fill in the blanks.

1. Describe facial and lingual innervation to the following teeth:
    a. maxillary first molar
    b. maxillary first premolar
    c. maxillary central incisor
    d. mandibular lateral incisor
    e. mandibular second premolar
    f. mandibular second molar

2. The longest cranial nerve is the_____ nerve.

3. The mandibular nerve supplies which of the following muscles?
    a. Buccinator
    b. Risorius
    c. Lateral pterygoid
    d. Genioglossus

4. Which cranial nerve supplies the sternocleidomastoid muscle?

5. List the nerves that form the pharyngeal plexus.

20

Arteries of the Head and Neck

INTERNAL CAROTID ARTERY
EXTERNAL CAROTID ARTERY
VEINS OF THE FACE

Objectives

- Describe the structures supplied by the internal carotid artery and branches of the external carotid artery.
- Describe blood supply to the maxillary and mandibular teeth.
- Describe the structures drained by the superficial and deep veins.
- Complete the worksheet at the end of the chapter.

The head and neck are supplied almost entirely by the *common carotid arteries*. On the left side, the common carotid ascends from the *arch of the aorta*. On the right side, it arises from the *brachiocephalic artery*. The common carotid arteries are found on the lateral sides of the neck beneath the sternocleidomastoid muscle (Figure 20-1). At the thyroid cartilage, the common carotid artery bifurcates into the *internal* and *external carotid arteries* (Figure 20-2).

INTERNAL CAROTID ARTERY

This artery does not supply the mouth. It enters the skull through the carotid canal and supplies the brain and eyes. There are no branches present in the neck (Figure 20-2).

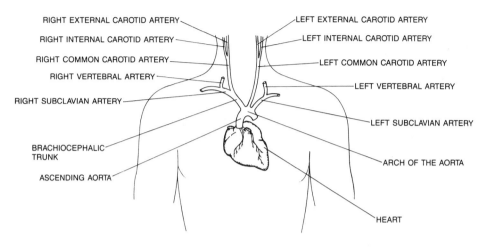

Figure 20-1 Origin of the carotid and vertebral arteries

EXTERNAL CAROTID ARTERY

This artery ascends in the neck to the angle of the mandible. It ends as it is crossed by the posterior belly of the digastric and stylohyoid muscles. Its branches cross the face and scalp. The external carotid has eight branches (Figures 20-2 and 20-3).

1. *Ascending pharyngeal:* This artery arises just above the bifurcation of the common carotid artery. It travels on the side of the pharynx on its way to the skull. It supplies the pharynx and its muscles (Figure 20-3).

2. *Superior thyroid:* This artery also arises from the bifurcation of the common carotid artery. It supplies the thyroid gland and associated muscles (Figure 20-3).

3. *Lingual:* The lingual artery arises at the level of the hyoid bone. It passes deep to the hyoglossus muscle and enters the base of the tongue. The lingual artery ends at the tip of the tongue. It has three branches.

   a. *Sublingual artery* — supplies the floor of the mouth, sublingual gland, mylohyoid muscle, and lingual gingiva.

   b. *Dorsal lingual artery* — supplies the back of the tongue, tonsils, soft palate, and epiglottis.

   c. *Deep lingual artery* — supplies the tip of the tongue along its inferior surface (Figures 20-3 and 20-4).

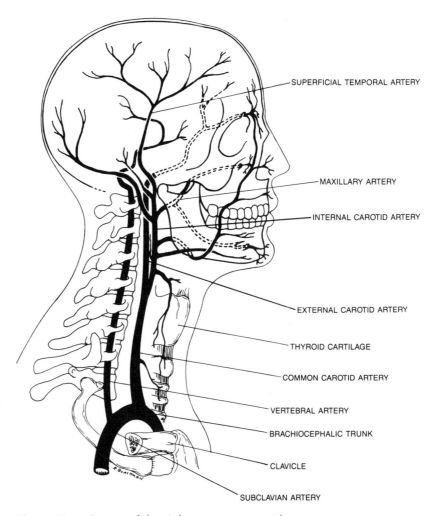

SUPERFICIAL TEMPORAL ARTERY

MAXILLARY ARTERY

INTERNAL CAROTID ARTERY

EXTERNAL CAROTID ARTERY

THYROID CARTILAGE

COMMON CAROTID ARTERY

VERTEBRAL ARTERY

BRACHIOCEPHALIC TRUNK

CLAVICLE

SUBCLAVIAN ARTERY

Figure 20-2 Course of the right common carotid artery

4. *Facial:* This arises just below the angle of the mandible. It passes close to the posterior belly of the digastric and stylohyoid muscles, and enters the submandibular gland. It travels lateral to the inferior border of the mandible, and then it turns and passes in front of the masseter muscle. After crossing the mandible, it travels obliquely across the face to the eye (Figure 20-3). It gives off six branches:

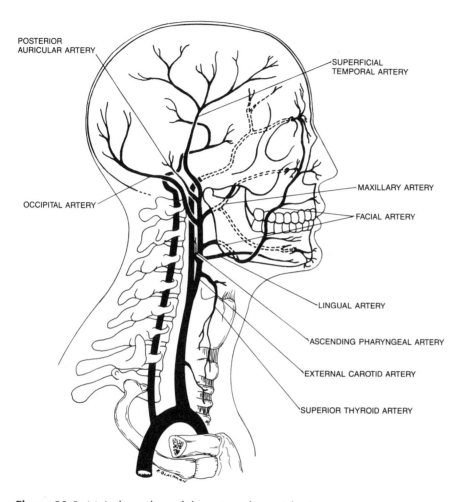

Figure 20-3 Main branches of the external carotid artery

a. *Ascending palatine artery* — supplies the soft palate, pharynx, pharyngeal muscles, and the tonsils. It arises at the beginning of the facial artery.

b. *Submental artery* — arises below the mandible and runs toward the chin. It supplies the sublingual and submandibular glands, mylohyoid muscle, and the anterior belly of the digastric muscle (Figure 20-5).

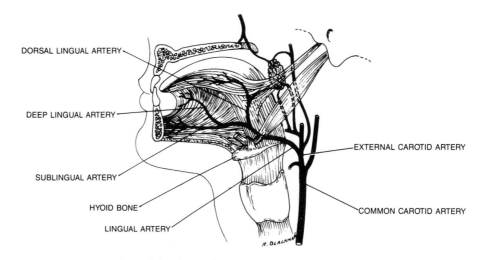

Figure 20-4 Branches of the lingual artery

c. *Inferior labial artery* — runs below the mouth deep to the orbicularis oris and supplies the lower lip and chin.

d. *Superior labial artery* — runs above the mouth and supplies the upper lip. The inferior and superior labial arteries arise at the corners of the mouth (Figure 20-5).

e. *Lateral nasal artery* — supplies the skin and muscles of the nose. It runs along the side of the nose.

f. *Angular artery* — the terminal branch of the facial artery. It supplies the eyelids and skin of the nose (Figure 20-5).

5. *Occipital:* This artery arises opposite the origin of the facial artery. It runs posteriorly toward the occipital area, and supplies the scalp and associated muscles, the sternocleidomastoid, and the muscles of the neck (Figure 20-3).

6. *Posterior auricular:* The posterior auricular artery arises opposite the ear, and travels behind the ear. It supplies the outer ear and associated scalp (Figure 20-3).

7. *Superficial temporal:* The superficial temporal artery and maxillary artery are the terminal branches of the external carotid artery. The superficial temporal artery travels through the parotid gland in front of the ear. Before the superficial artery emerges from the parotid gland, it gives off the *transverse facial artery* which supplies the masseter muscle and parotid

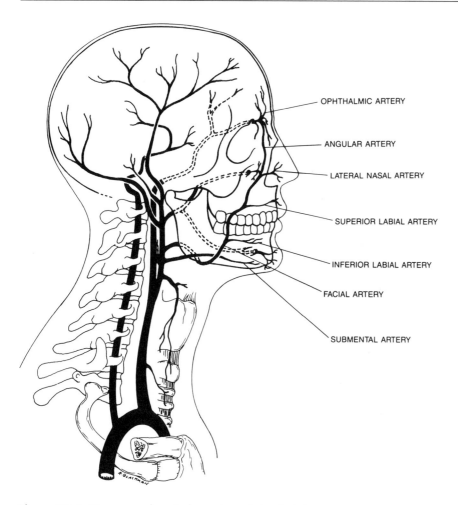

OPHTHALMIC ARTERY

ANGULAR ARTERY

LATERAL NASAL ARTERY

SUPERIOR LABIAL ARTERY

INFERIOR LABIAL ARTERY

FACIAL ARTERY

SUBMENTAL ARTERY

Figure 20-5 Course and main branches of the facial artery

gland. *Auricular* branches travel to the ear, and a *middle temporal* branch supplies the temporalis muscle (Figures 20-2 and 20-3).

8. *Maxillary:* The maxillary artery is the larger of the two terminal branches of the external carotid. It arises from the external carotid artery at the neck of the mandible. It passes between the mandible and sphenomandibular ligament, close to the lateral pterygoid muscle, on its way to the pterygopalatine fossa. It supplies facial structures and is divided into three sections: *mandibular, pterygoid,* and *pterygopalatine* (Figure 20-6).

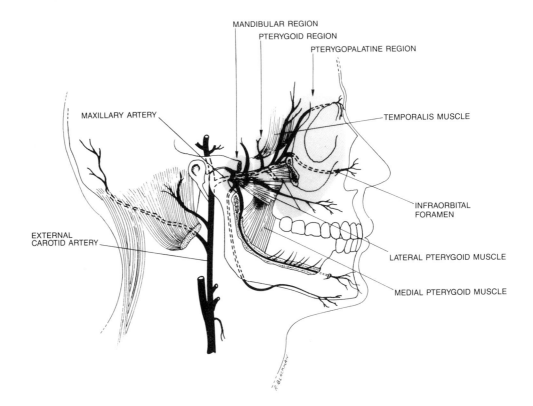

Figure 20-6 The three regions of the maxillary artery

Mandibular Section

This section is located behind the neck of the mandible. There are five branches found here.

1. *Deep auricular artery* — supplies the temporomandibular joint, external acoustic meatus, and the tympanic membrane (Figure 20-7).

2. *Anterior tympanic artery* — supplies the inside of the tympanic membrane (Figure 20-7).

3. *Inferior alveolar artery* — travels with the inferior alveolar nerve and enters the mandibular foramen. This artery supplies the mandibular molar and premolar teeth (Figure 20-7).

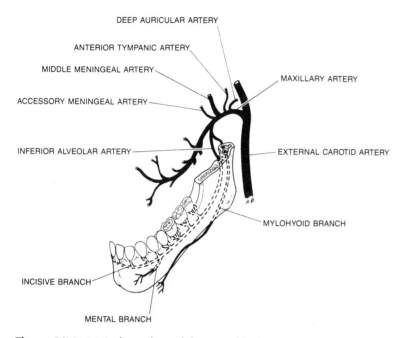

Figure 20-7 Main branches of the mandibular area of the maxillary artery

Before the inferior alveolar artery enters the mandibular foramen, it gives off a branch, the *mylohyoid artery*, which travels in the mylohyoid groove to supply the mylohyoid muscle. A *lingual branch* is also given off which aids in supplying the tongue. The inferior alveolar artery travels in the mandibular canal until it reaches the mental foramen at which point it branches into the *mental artery* and *incisive artery*. The mental artery supplies the chin, while the incisive artery supplies the mandibular anterior teeth together with the incisive artery of the opposite side. *Dental branches* enter through the apical foramen to supply the pulp. Dental branches correspond to the number of roots.

4. *Middle meningeal artery* — ascends between the lateral pterygoid muscle and the sphenomandibular ligament, and between the roots of the auriculotemporal nerve. It enters the cranium through the foramen spinosum to supply the dura mater and cranium (Figure 20-7).

5. *Accessory meningeal artery* — travels through the foramen ovale to supply the dura mater and trigeminal ganglion (Figure 20-7).

Pterygoid Section

This section is located in the infratemporal fossa (Figure 20-6). It has six branches.

> **1 & 2.** *Posterior and anterior deep temporal arteries* — supply the temporalis muscle.
>
> **3.** *Masseteric artery* — supplies the masseter muscle.
>
> **4 & 5.** *Medial and lateral pterygoid arteries* — supply the medial and lateral pterygoid muscles.
>
> **6.** *Buccal artery* — supplies the buccinator muscle and the cheek.

Pterygopalatine Section

This section is located in the pterygopalatine fossa. The maxillary artery ends around the infraorbital area. There are six branches found here.

> **1.** *Posterior superior alveolar artery* — travels across the maxilla with the posterior superior alveolar nerve. Branches supply the maxillary molar teeth, maxillary sinus, and associated gingiva (Figure 20-8).

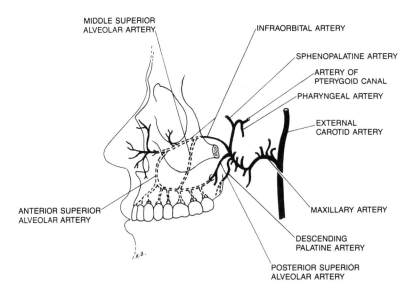

Figure 20-8 Main branches of the pterygopalatine region of the maxillary artery

2. *Infraorbital artery* — emerges onto the face through the infraorbital foramen. A *middle superior alveolar branch* supplies the maxillary pre-molar teeth. An *anterior superior branch* supplies the maxillary incisors and canine teeth. The lacrimal sacs and lower eyelids are supplied by the *palpebral branches. Labial branches* supply the upper lip, while *nasal branches* supply the nose (Figure 20-8).

3. *Greater palatine artery* — emerges from the greater palatine foramen to supply the gingiva, palatine glands, and the roof of the mouth. The *lesser palatine branch* emerges from the lesser palatine foramen to supply the tonsils and soft palate.

4. *Artery of the pterygoid canal* — arises in the pterygopalatine fossa and enters the pterygoid canal. It supplies the upper part of the pharynx, auditory tube, and tympanic cavity (Figure 20-8).

5. *Pharyngeal artery* — runs posteriorly to supply the sphenoid sinus, upper part of the pharynx, and auditory tube (Figure 20-8).

6. *Sphenopalatine artery* — enters the nasal cavity through the sphenopalatine foramen. It divides into two branches (Figure 20-8):

   a. *Posterior lateral nasal artery* — aids in supplying the frontal, maxillary, ethmoid, and sphenoid sinuses.

   b. *Posterior septal artery* — supplies the nasal septum. One branch, the *nasopalatine artery*, travels to the incisive foramen where it joins with the greater palatine artery.

VEINS OF THE FACE

The veins of the face usually travel with arteries and have similar names. Veins are commonly divided into a superficial and a deep group. Variations in venous drainage are common. Facial veins do not have valves, so there is a potential danger of infection to the brain.

Superficial Veins

The *facial* and *superficial temporal* veins drain facial structures. The facial vein becomes the *angular* vein after it passes the upper lip. The facial vein has several branches from the nose, lips, eye, submental, and submandibular regions.

The superficial temporal vein joins the *maxillary* vein to form the *retromandibular vein* (Figure 20-9). This vein drains the regions of the maxillary and superficial temporal arteries.

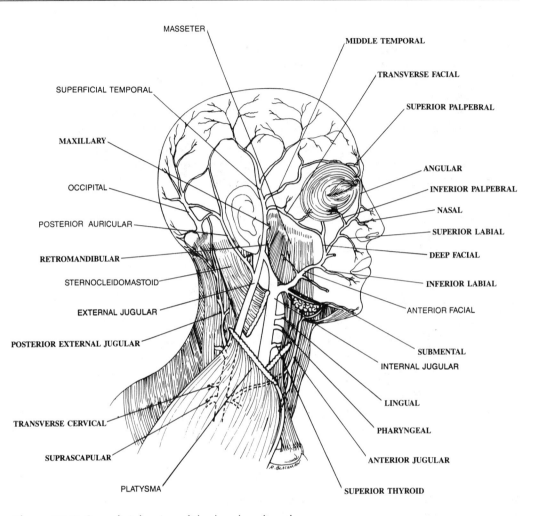

Figure 20-9 Superficial veins of the head and neck

The *common facial* vein is the union of the facial and retromandibular veins. It then enters the *internal jugular* vein (Figure 20-10). The internal jugular vein empties into the *brachiocephalic* vein. The right and left *brachiocephalic* veins join and form the *superior vena cava* which drains into the heart.

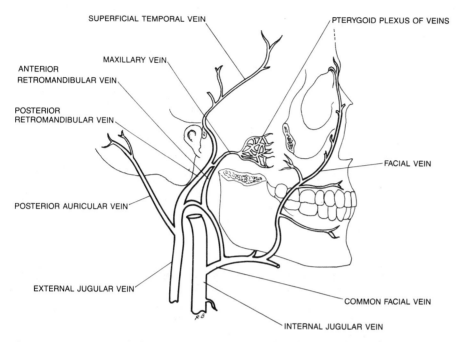

Figure 20-10 General drainage areas of internal and external jugular veins

Deep Veins

Pterygoid plexus is a collection of veins located between the temporalis and lateral pterygoid muscles and between the lateral and medial pterygoids. Structures that drain into this plexus include: muscles of mastication, buccinator, nose, palate, and the teeth. The *maxillary* vein drains the pterygoid plexus (Figures 20-10 and 20-11).

SUMMARY

The head and neck are supplied almost entirely by the common carotid arteries. These are divided into three groups in the head and neck: (1) the *internal carotid artery*, which supplies the brain and eye; (2) the *external carotid artery*, which supplies the mouth and head and includes eight branches — ascending pharyngeal, superior thyroid, lingual, facial, occipital, posterior auricular, superficial temporal, and maxillary; and (3) the *veins of the face*, which generally travel with the arteries and are divided into superficial and deep veins.

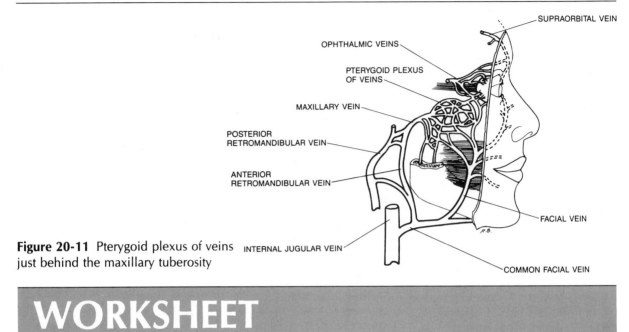

Figure 20-11 Pterygoid plexus of veins just behind the maxillary tuberosity

WORKSHEET

A. Trace a drop of blood from the heart on both sides of the body to the:
   a. maxillary anteriors
   b. mandibular premolars
   c. muscles of mastication

B. Complete the following figures.

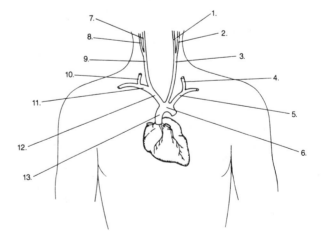

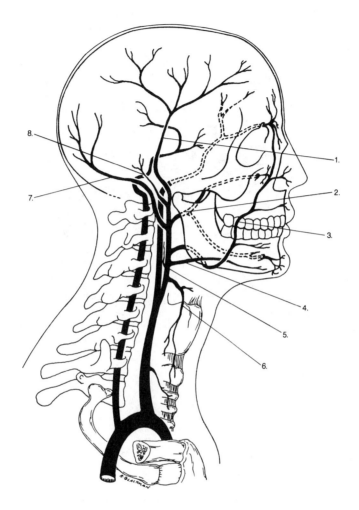

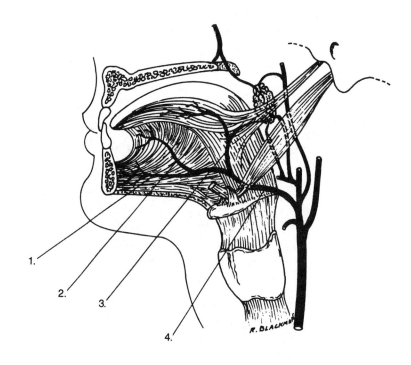

1.

2.

3.

4.

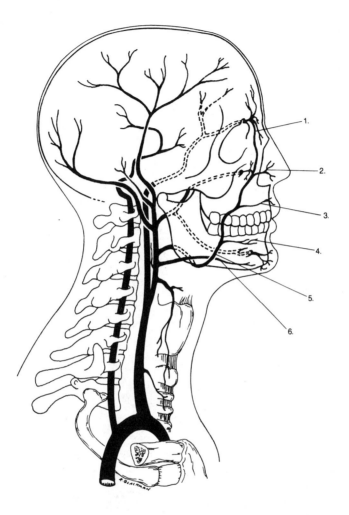

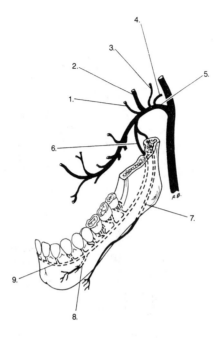

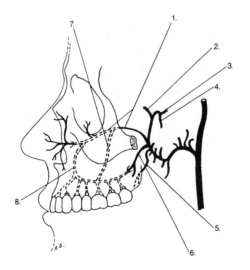

C. Answer the following questions.

1. What branch of the common carotid artery supplies the brain?

2. What branch of the external carotid artery supplies the teeth?

3. What artery supplies the following teeth:
   a. mandibular molars
   b. maxillary molars
   c. mandibular anteriors
   d. maxillary premolars

4. What deep vein drains the teeth?

5. What section of the maxillary artery supplies the muscles of mastication?

21

Salivary Glands

MAJOR SALIVARY GLANDS
MINOR SALIVARY GLANDS

Objectives

- Differentiate between major and minor salivary glands.
- Describe the location of the major and minor salivary glands.
- Identify the duct for each major salivary gland.
- Classify each of the major and minor salivary glands according to its secretion.
- Complete the worksheet at the end of the chapter.

In the oral cavity, there are *major* and *minor* salivary glands. The three pairs of major salivary glands are the *parotid, submandibular,* and *sublingual.* Minor salivary glands may be located through the mouth.

MAJOR SALIVARY GLANDS

Parotid Gland

The parotid gland is the largest of the three major salivary glands. It is located on the side of the face, below and in front of the ear and behind the ramus. It terminates at the zygomatic arch in front of the ear and reaches down the masseter muscle. It extends inward to the pharyngeal wall. The duct for this gland is known as *Stensen's duct,* which crosses the masseter and buccinator muscles to enter the oral cavity

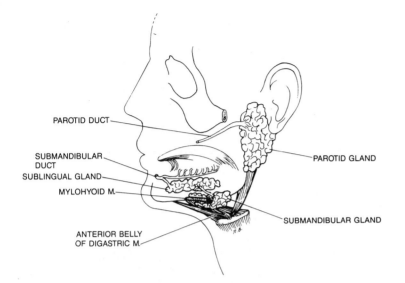

Figure 21-1 Locations and ducts of the major salivary glands

opposite the maxillary second molar. Stensen's duct is covered by the *parotid papilla*, a small papilla extending from the cheek mucosa opposite the maxillary second molar (Figures 21-1 and 21-2).

The parotid gland is surrounded by a fibrous capsule. Several structures, such as the superficial temporal artery, retromandibular vein, and the facial nerve pierce the gland and travel within it. Saliva produced by the parotid gland is purely serous. Mumps is a viral infection of this gland.

Submandibular Gland

The submandibular gland is about the size of a walnut. It is located in the submandibular triangle which is in front of and underneath the inferior border of the mandible (Figures 21-1, 21-2, and 21-3). A small part extends to the mylohyoid muscle and lies deep to it. The remainder of the gland is located superficially to the mylohyoid muscle. The two divisions are connected. Its duct is known as *Wharton's duct*, which opens into the mouth at the sublingual caruncle.

A capsule encloses this gland. The facial artery is embedded in the submandibular gland. Saliva produced by this gland is mixed, 80% serous, 20% mucous. Serous secretions are thin and watery, while mucous production is thick and viscous.

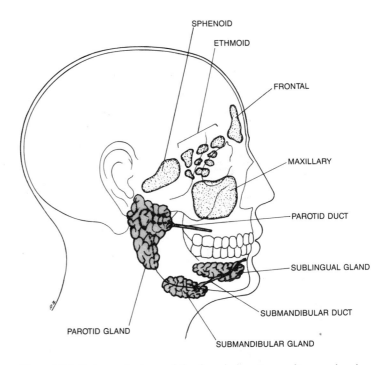

SPHENOID

ETHMOID

FRONTAL

MAXILLARY

PAROTID DUCT

SUBLINGUAL GLAND

SUBMANDIBULAR DUCT

PAROTID GLAND

SUBMANDIBULAR GLAND

Figure 21-2 Lateral view of the head showing salivary glands

Sublingual Gland

The sublingual gland is the smallest of the major salivary glands. It is located beneath the sublingual mucosa in the floor of the mouth. This gland rests on the mylohyoid muscle and its projection forms the sublingual fold or *plica sublingualis* along the floor of the mouth. It has several small ducts, 8 to 20 in number, known as the *ducts of Rivinus*. These small ducts empty onto the sublingual fold. It has one major duct, *Bartholin's duct*, which opens along with Wharton's duct at the sublingual caruncle (Figures 21-1, 21-2, and 21-3).

The sublingual gland is not encapsulated. It secretes a mixed saliva, but it is primarily a mucous secretion.

MINOR SALIVARY GLANDS

The minor salivary glands are small glands with short ducts that open directly into the mouth. Saliva secreted by these glands is usually mixed.

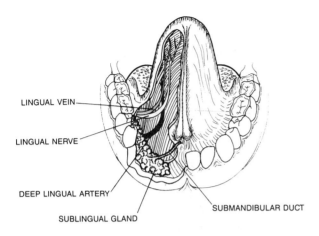

LINGUAL VEIN

LINGUAL NERVE

DEEP LINGUAL ARTERY

SUBLINGUAL GLAND

SUBMANDIBULAR DUCT

Figure 21-3 Inferior surface of the tongue

Labial Glands

These glands are found in the submucosa of the lips. They are numerous at the midline and have small ducts that open directly onto the lip mucosa. These are mixed glands, primarily mucous (Figure 21-4).

Buccal Glands

The buccal glands are located in the cheek. They are very similar to the labial glands.

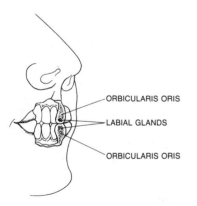

ORBICULARIS ORIS

LABIAL GLANDS

ORBICULARIS ORIS

Figure 21-4 Labial glands

Palatine Glands

These glands are found on the posterior one-third of the palate and on the soft palate. The opening of these ducts may be large and visible. They are pure mucous in secretion (Figure 21-5).

Lingual Glands

The lingual glands can be divided into three groups:

The *anterior lingual glands,* glands of the Blandin and Nuhn, are located at the apex of the tongue. The ducts empty onto the ventral surface of the tongue. They are mainly mucous in nature.

The *lingual glands of Von Ebner* are found beneath the vallate papillae. Their ducts open into the trough of the papillae. They are purely serous.

The *posterior lingual glands* can be found near the lingual tonsils on the posterior one-third of the tongue. They are purely mucous.

SUMMARY

The oral cavity is supplied by major and minor salivary glands. The major salivary glands include (1) the *parotid,* which is located in front of the ear and supplies the mouth with serous saliva; (2) the *submandibular,* which is located in front of and underneath the mandible and supplies the mouth with mixed saliva; (3) the *sublingual,* which is located beneath the sublingual mucosa in the floor of the mouth and supplies the mouth with mixed saliva, primarily mucous.

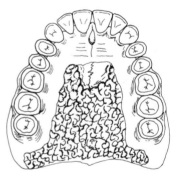

Figure 21-5 Palatine glands

   The minor salivary glands include (1) the *labial*, which are located in the lip submucosa and supply the mouth with saliva that is primarily mucous; (2) the *buccal*, which is located in the buccal mucosa and supplies the mouth with saliva that is primarily mucous; (3) the *palatine*, which is located in the lip submucosa and supplies the mouth with saliva that is purely mucous; (4) the *lingual*, which are divided into three groups — the anterior lingual glands (Blandin and Nuhn), the lingual glands of Von Ebner, and the posterior lingual glands.

WORKSHEET

A. Place a check under the correct response.

SALIVARY GLAND	SEROUS	MUCOUS	MIXED
Parotid			
Submandibular			
Sublingual			
Labial			
Buccal			
Palatine			
Anterior Lingual			
Lingual glands of Von Ebner Posterior Lingual			

B. Complete the following figure.

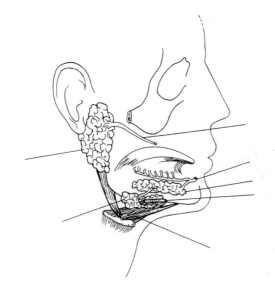

C. Answer the following questions and fill in the blanks.

1. Fill in the chart.

SALIVARY GLAND	DUCT
Parotid	
Submandibular	
Sublingual	

2. What duct is covered by the parotid papilla?

3. What two ducts open at the sublingual caruncle?

4. What cranial nerve is found within the parotid gland?

5. The lingual glands of Von Ebner are located beneath the _____ papillae.

22

Clinical Considerations

Objectives

By the completion of this chapter the material studied in Chapters 1 through 21 can be applied in a clinical situation. It is necessary for the reader to have a dental chair, adequate light, a dental mirror, an explorer, and a periodontal probe.

Although the theory can be learned from the readings, it is often easier to remember details by observing them directly as they would be seen from a clinical point of view. It is also important to realize that the structures emphasized in the text are those that will relate to use of instruments, preventive care, or restorative dentistry; emphasis is on the relationship of form to function. It is important to see how the content of the chapters can be useful to the dental auxiliary.

CHAPTER 1: NOMENCLATURE

Before completing the following exercises, observe the shapes of the teeth, noticing how they differ. Have your patient open and close the teeth, noticing the manner in which they interdigitate.

1. Describe the shapes of the teeth and relate this to their specific function.

   a. incisors —

   b. canines —

   c. premolars —

   d. molars —

262

2. Observe the incisal edges and occlusal surfaces. Record those teeth that have attrition and the reason you feel this occurred.

3. Observe the cervix, mesial and distal surfaces, and occlusal surface of posterior teeth. How do you think the curvatures and shapes of these surfaces affect food or deposit retention?

4. Try to visualize your various scalers. How do the shapes of the teeth (anterior and posterior; mesial and distal) affect the adaptation of curets, sickles, or hoes?

CHAPTER 2: STRUCTURES OF THE ORAL CAVITY

Review all the structures of the oral cavity so that you will be able to recognize the normal and any deviation from it.

For each structure listed, provide the following information:

- its precise location in the oral cavity
- its clinical appearance (size, shape, color, texture)
- its comparison to the normal

Using the above information as a guide, complete your observations.

1. Vermillion area: Is there crackling? Note any sores. What is the variation in coloring?

2. Philtrum: Note the depth of concavity. How does this affect one's appearance?

3. Maxillary tuberosity: Is this a large projection? What is the condition of the tissue?

4. Retromolar area: Is this mucosa about the same consistency as the buccal mucosa? How large an area is this?

5. Labial frenum: About how many millimeters is this small extension of tissue? Does it extend onto the attached gingiva?

6. Lingual frenum: What is the extent of its length? Is it raised or flat?

7. Buccal frenum: In what position must the jaws be before this can be observed? Which posterior teeth lie adjacent to this?

8. Incisive papilla: Is it raised, flat, inflamed?

9. Palatine rugae: Are they raised or flat? How many pairs are observed?

10. Palatine raphe: How far does this extend along the palate? Is it clearly observed?

11. Fovea palatinus: Are they on the hard or soft palate? What is their depth?

12. Pillars of fauces: Provide another name for the anterior and posterior pillar. What are the limits?

13. Palatine tonsils: Are they present? Describe their position and condition.

14. Uvula: Is it inflamed? What is the length?

15. Tongue: Observe the size and papilla: Is it coated?

16. Sublingual caruncles: Can you see the duct openings? Describe what the duct openings are like. How high are the caruncles?

17. Buccal mucosa: Is it consistently pink and soft?

18. Stenson's papilla: Which posterior tooth is adjacent to this? Can the opening to the duct be seen?

CHAPTER 3: THE TOOTH AND ITS SURROUNDING STRUCTURES

1. Observe the crowns of the teeth. Record those teeth where the clinical crown is greater than the anatomical crown.

2. Using the chart below, draw the height of the free gingiva of the maxillary molars. This is drawn on both the buccal and lingual surfaces.

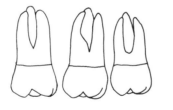

BUCCAL

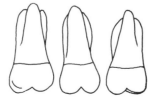

LINGUAL

3. With an explorer, locate the cervical line (CEJ) of the right molars.

    a. Is the cervical line clinically visible on all teeth?

    b. Is the clinical crown larger or smaller than the anatomical crown?

4. Observe the gingiva. Locate and describe the following sections as they appear in the oral cavity:

    a. Marginal (free) gingiva

    b. Interdental papilla

    c. Attached gingiva

    d. Muco-gingival line

    e. Alveolar mucosa

5. Use a periodontal probe to feel the depth and continuity of the gingival sulcus around teeth #6–8 and #30.

    a. What is the approximate depth of a normal sulcus? _____

    b. What is the sulcus depth of the teeth just explored?

      #6 _____ #7 _____ #8 _____ #30 _____

6. Observe the occlusal surfaces and note that they are not smooth. They have pits and grooves. Follow these grooves, gently, with an explorer. If the explorer sticks, record the tooth and surface below.

CHAPTER 4: NUMBERING SYSTEMS

1. Observe the teeth in each quadrant and record those that are missing by using the following numbering systems.
    a. Universal Numbering System
    b. Palmer's Notation
    c. F.D.I.

2. Observe the maxillary first molar. Record its antagonist(s) by using the Universal Numbering System.

3. Record the left premolars using Palmer's Notation. Using the same recording methods, note the deciduous teeth that precede the premolars.

4. Using the Universal Numbering System, record the third tooth from the midline and the fourth tooth from the midline, both maxillary and mandibular. Are these the same teeth in the permanent and deciduous dentition?

5. Record the first permanent tooth to erupt. _____

6. Which tooth replaces #18d? _____

7. Compare the crowns of #9 and #10.

CHAPTERS 5 through 7: (SECTION TWO-PERMANENT ANTERIOR TEETH)

General Observations

1. Observe the antagonist(s) of all anterior teeth. Record the antagonist(s) of the following teeth:
   a. Maxillary central incisor
   b. Mandibular central incisor
   c. Mandibular canine

2. Record the name of the smallest anterior tooth. Observe this tooth in the oral cavity. What is the approximate difference in width (mm) from both its proximal teeth?

3. Which anterior tooth is the widest mesio-distally? Observe it in the oral cavity and record the difference in width (mm) with the proximal tooth that sits distally.

4. Observe all the incisors. Which has the most rounded disto-incisal angle?

5. Using the perioprobe, measure the length of the crowns.

   a. Compare the length of the maxillary central to the mandibular central incisor; the maxillary central to the maxillary lateral incisor.

   b. Which anterior tooth is the longest?

6. Observe all the incisal edges. Are mamelons present?

7. Record those incisors that have labial depressions.

8. Observe all the canines. Which buccal lobe forms the cusp tip? Which forms the buccal ridge?

9. Observe the cingulum of all anterior teeth. Which are the most highly developed?

10. Compare the fossa of all anterior teeth. Are irregularities present? Record your observations. What clinical significance would this have?

11. After observing the crowns of all anterior teeth, describe how the contours will affect deposit accumulation.

12. Describe which scalers will best adapt to anterior teeth and why. Are there any anatomical considerations that require special consideration while scaling? While polishing?

CHAPTERS 8 through 12 (SECTION THREE - PERMANENT POSTERIOR TEETH)

Premolars

1. Observe the buccal surfaces of both maxillary and mandibular premolars. Is there any clear way to differentiate them?

2. Observe the premolars from the occlusal or lingual surfaces. Now they should be more easily identified by cusps and grooves. Record those that have a lingual groove. Make a note if it contains a restoration.

3. Do the mandibular second premolars in this mouth have two or three cusps?

4. Your clinical observations will not give you a clue to the number of roots. Do premolars have one or two roots? If you were to scale the root surfaces, would the number of roots require special consideration?

5. Record the premolar that occludes with a molar. What is the molar to premolar cusp relationship?

6. Observe the grooves of all premolars and any restorations that may be present. Notice the number of supplementary grooves in each tooth. How would this affect the type of patient education needed?

Molars

1. Observe the mandibular first molar to see if there is a pit or concave area at the base of the mesio-buccal groove.

2. Use your explorer to examine the cervical line on all molars. Record your observations as to smoothness, concave areas, etc.

3. Examine the molar area for gingival recession. How far, apically, would you expect to find the root furcation?

4. Examine the occlusal surfaces of all the right, or left, molars with an explorer. Record all deep grooves and pits:

Mandibular M_1 Maxillary M_1

M_2 M_2

M_3 M_3

If there is a restoration in the occlusal, place an X on the paper.

5. Examine the contour of the crowns. Adapt various scalers (curet, sickle, hoe) to determine which best fits the shape of the tooth. Record your observations.

CHAPTER 13: DECIDUOUS DENTITION

1. Observe the deciduous molars. Which deciduous molar resembles the first permanent molar?

2. Observe the spacing between the deciduous teeth. Record those areas where there is no spacing. How could this affect the position of the permanent teeth?

3. Do the shapes of the deciduous crowns resemble their permanent counterparts? Record those that do not.

4. Examine the occlusal surfaces with an explorer and record any deep pit or grooves. Do deciduous teeth require the same oral hygiene as permanent teeth?

5. Have the patient occlude and record the antagonists of the maxillary second molar; mandibular central incisor.

6. After observing the convexities and concavities of the anterior teeth, comment on the positioning of a toothbrush or engine polisher when cleaning these teeth.

CHAPTERS 15 and 16: OCCLUSION

1. Observe the patient's profile and record.

2. Establish centric occlusion by asking your patient to close the posterior teeth.
   a. Describe the normal relationship of the molars.

   b. Which of the following best describes your patient's molar relationship?
   Class I _____
   Class II _____
   Class III _____

   c. Describe any other malrelationships that are observed.

3. Observe the contact areas of all teeth and record where there is no contact. How does this affect occlusion?

4. Observe the interdental papilla of all teeth and record those areas where it does not reach the contact area. List some of the causes and effects of this.

SUMMARY

Actual involvement in a project helps to retain the knowledge of the material, but these exercises will also provide an opportunity to see how the subject matter applies to a clinical situation.

APPENDIXES

APPENDIX A

DEVELOPMENT OF THE TEETH

Table A-1. Deciduous Dentition

	FORMATION OF THE ENAMEL ORGAN (WEEKS IN UTERO)	BEGINNING OF CALCIFICATION (MONTHS IN UTERO)	CROWN COMPLETION (MONTHS)	ERUPTION (MONTHS)	ROOT COMPLETION (YEARS)
MAXILLARY					
Central Incisor	10	3-4	4	7½	1½-2
Lateral Incisor	12	4½	5	8	1½-2
Canine	14	5¼	9	16-20	2½-3
First Molar	13-14	5	6	12-16	2-2½
Second Molar	15-16	6	10-12	20-30	3
MANDIBULAR					
Central Incisor	11	4½	4	6½	1½-2
Lateral Incisor	12	4½	4¼	7	1½-2
Canine	14	5	9	16-20	2½-3
First Molar	13-14	5	6	12-16	2-2½
Second Molar	15-16	6	10-12	20-30	3

Table A-2. Permanent Dentition

	FORMATION OF THE ENAMEL ORGAN (MONTHS IN UTERO*)	BEGINNING OF CALCIFICATION	CROWN COMPLETION (YEARS)	ERUPTION (YEARS)	ROOT COMPLETION (YEARS)
MAXILLARY					
Central Incisor	7	3-4 mo	4-5	7-8	10
Lateral Incisor	7	10 mo	4-5	8-9	11
Canine	7	4-5 mo	6-7	11-12	13-15
First Premolar	7	1½-1 yr	5-6	10-11	12-13
Second Premolar	7	2-2½ yr	6-7	10-12	12-14
First Molar	5½	Birth	2½-3	6-7	9-10
Second Molar	6 mo after birth	2½-3 yr	7-8	12-13	14-15
Third Molar	6 yr after birth	7-9 yr	12-16	17-21	18-25
MANDIBULAR					
Central Incisor	7	3-4 mo	4-5	6-7	9
Lateral Incisor	7	3-4 mo	4-5	7-8	10
Canine	7	4-5 mo	6-7	9-10	12-14
First Premolar	7	1¼-2 yr	5-6	10-12	12-13
Second Premolar	7	2¼-2½ yr	6-7	11-12	13-14
First Molar	5½	Birth	2½-3	6-7	9-10
Second Molar	6 mo after birth	2½-3 yr	7-8	11-13	14-15
Third Molar	6 yr after birth	8-10 yr	12-16	17-21	18-25

*Except where noted

Table A-3. Chronology of the Human Dentition*

		BEGINNING OF CALCIFICATION	CROWN COMPLETION	ERUPTION	ROOT COMPLETION
DECIDUOUS DENTITION					
Upper jaw	Central incisor	3-4 mo in utero	4 mo	7½ mo	1½-2 yr
	Lateral incisor	4½ mo in utero	5 mo	8 mo	1½-2 yr
	Canine	5¼ mo in utero	9 mo	16-20 mo	2½-3 yr
	First molar	5 mo in utero	6 mo	12-16 mo	2-2½ yr
	Second molar	6 mo in utero	10-12 mo	20-30 mo	3 yr
Lower jaw	Central incisor	4½ mo in utero	4 mo	6½ mo	1½-2 yr
	Lateral incisor	4½ mo in utero	4¼ mo	7 mo	1½-2 yr
	Canine	5 mo in utero	9 mo	16-20 mo	2½-3 yr
	First molar	5 mo in utero	6 mo	12-16 mo	2-2½ yr
	Second molar	6 mo in utero	10-12 mo	20-30 mo	3 yr
PERMANENT DENTITION					
Upper jaw	Central incisor	3-4 mo	4-5 yr	7-8 yr	10 yr
	Lateral incisor	10 mo	4-5 yr	8-9 yr	11 yr
	Canine	4-5 mo	6-7 yr	11-12 yr	13-15 yr
	First premolar	1¼-1½ yr	5-6 yr	10-11 yr	12-13 yr
	Second premolar	2-2¼ yr	6-7 yr	10-12 yr	12-14 yr
	First molar	At birth	2½-3 yr	6-7 yr	9-10 yr
	Second molar	2½-3 yr	7-8 yr	12-13 yr	14-16 yr
	Third molar	7-9 yr	12-16 yr	17-21 yr	18-25 yr
Lower jaw	Central incisor	3-4 mo	4-5 yr	6-7 yr	9 yr
	Lateral incisor	3-4 mo	4-5 yr	7-8 yr	10 yr
	Canine	4-5 mo	6-7 yr	9-10 yr	12-14 yr
	First premolar	1¼-2 yr	5-6 yr	10-12 yr	12-13 yr
	Second premolar	2¼-2½ yr	6-7 yr	11-12 yr	13-14 yr
	First molar	At birth	2½-3 yr	6-7 yr	9-10 yr
	Second molar	2½-3 yr	7-8 yr	11-13 yr	14-15 yr
	Third molar	8-10 yr	12-16 yr	17-21 yr	18-25 yr

*From R. Wheeler, *Textbook of Dental Anatomy and Physiology* (Philadelphia: W.B. Saunders, 1965), 30. Copyright by the American Dental Association. Reprinted by permission.

APPENDIX B

MEASUREMENTS OF THE TEETH

MAXILLARY TEETH	LENGTH OF CROWN	LENGTH OF ROOT	MESIO-DISTAL DIAM-ETER OF CROWN†	MESIO-DISTAL DIAM-ETER AT CERVIX	LABIO- OR BUCCO-LINGUAL DIAM-ETER	LABIO- OR BUCCO-LINGUAL DIAM-ETER AT CERVIX	CURVA-TURE OF CERVICAL LINE — MESIAL	CURVA-TURE OF CERVICAL LINE — DISTAL
Central Incisor	10.5	13.0	8.5	7.0	7.0	6.0	3.5	2.5
Lateral Incisor	9.0	13.0	6.5	5.0	6.0	5.0	3.0	2.0
Canine	10.0	17.0	7.5	5.5	8.0	7.0	2.5	1.5
1st Premolar	8.5	14.0	7.0	5.0	9.0	8.0	1.0	0.0
2d Premolar	8.5	14.0	7.0	5.0	9.0	8.0	1.0	0.0
First Molar	7.5	b 12 l 13	10.0	8.0	11.0	10.0	1.0	0.0
Second Molar	7.0	b 11 l 12	9.0	7.0	11.0	10.0	1.0	0.0
Third Molar	6.5	11.0	8.5	6.5	10.0	9.5	1.0	0.0

MANDIBULAR TEETH	LENGTH OF CROWN	LENGTH OF ROOT	MESIO-DISTAL DIAM-ETER AT CROWN†	MESIO-DISTAL DIAM-ETER AT CERVIX	LABIO- OR BUCCO-LINGUAL DIAM-ETER	LABIO- OR BUCCO LINGUAL DIAM-ETER AT CERVIX	CURVA-TURE OF CERVICAL LINE — MESIAL	CURVA-TURE OF CERVICAL LINE — DISTAL
Central Incisor	9.0†	12.5	5.0	3.5	6.0	5.3	3.0	2.0
Lateral Incisor	9.5†	14.0	5.5	4.0	6.5	5.8	3.0	2.0
Canine	11.0	16.0	7.0	5.5	7.5	7.0	2.5	1.0
1st Premolar	8.5	14.0	7.0	5.0	7.5	6.5	1.0	0.0
2d Premolar	8.0	14.5	7.0	5.0	8.0	7.0	1.0	0.0
First Molar	7.5	14.0	11.0	9.0	10.5	9.0	1.0	0.0
Second Molar	7.0	13.0	10.5	8.0	10.0	9.0	1.0	0.0
Third Molar	7.0	11.0	10.0	7.5	9.5	9.0	1.0	0.0

From Ash: *Wheeler's Dental Anatomy, Physiology and Occlusion,*
6th Edition (W.B. Saunders, 1984).

†In millimeters

APPENDIX C

DIRECTIONS FOR DRAWING AND CARVING TEETH

DRAWING TEETH

1. Draw a base line representing the incisal or occlusal edge.
2. Measure the height of the crown and root; place a mark for each on the paper.
3. Draw a midline, for symmetry.
4. Divide the crown into thirds.
5. Place an X at the crest of curvatures.
6. Using the widest measurement, place the marks in the appropriate third. Be sure the midline is used.
7. Place X's in the cervical third at the narrowest points.
8. Connect the X's to conform with the shape of the crown as described in the reading.
9. Draw the root.
10. Draw specific anatomy as described in the reading. If the cingulum occupies one third of the lingual, be sure that it is drawn in the appropriate space and with the correct curvatures.

Include other structures such as fossae, ridges, grooves.

CARVING OCCLUSAL SURFACES

1. Review the size and shape of the surface.
2. Review and draw the groove pattern.
3. Mark the location of the grooves on the waxed surface.
4. Carve an inclined plane toward the central groove.
5. Carve inclined planes toward the fossae.
6. Check the height of the triangular ridges and marginal ridges.
7. Recarve grooves.
8. Smooth and finish the surface.

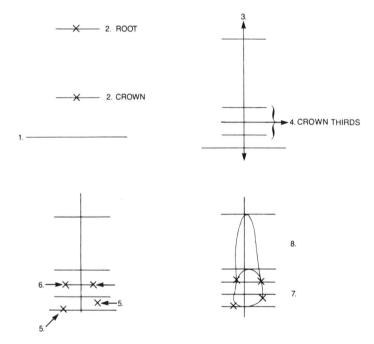

Glossary

ACTIVE ERUPTION — the emergence of the tooth from its position in the jaw to its position in occlusion.

AFFERENT — nerves that carry sensory messages toward the brain.

ALIGNMENT — arranged in a row or a line.

ALVEOLAR CREST — the highest portion of alveolar bone.

ALVEOLAR EMINENCE — outline of the root on the facial portion of the bone.

ALVEOLAR PROCESS — that portion of the maxilla or mandible that surrounds the root of the teeth.

ALVEOLUS — a socket in the bone in which the tooth sits.

ANATOMICAL CROWN — the portion of the tooth that is covered with enamel.

ANOMALY — a deviation from the normal.

ANTAGONIST — a structure that opposes or counteracts another structure; in the oral cavity, the teeth that meet those in the opposite jaw.

ANTERIOR — situated in front of.

APEX — a pointed extremity of a structure.

APICAL FORAMEN — an aperture in the apex of the root.

APPOSITION — laying down of, or addition of.

ARCH — a curvature; both the maxillary and mandibular teeth are positioned in an arch formation.

ATTRITION — wearing away by normal use (chewing, biting, etc.).

AXON — the process that carries impulses away from the cell body.

BIFURCATION — having two branches; forking into two parts.

BILATERAL — both sides.

BUCCAL — relating to the cheek.

CALCIFICATION — process of hardening by the deposit of calcium salts.

CANAL — a large opening through a bone.

CENTRIC OCCLUSION — the relationship of the occlusal surfaces of one arch to those in the opposing arch at physical rest position.

CENTRIC RELATION — the relationship of the maxillary arch to the mandibular arch when the condyle is in its most retruded position.

CERVICAL — relating to the cervix or neck of the tooth.

CERVIX — the neck of the tooth; the area where the crown joins the root or enamel joins the cementum.

CINGULUM — an eminence or raised area on the lingual surface of the anterior teeth resulting from the lingual lobe formation.

CLINICAL CROWN — that portion of the tooth visible in the mouth; it extends from the occlusal or incisal edge to the crest of the free gingiva.

CONCAVE — curving inward; a depression.

CONTACT AREA — that portion of the proximal surface of a tooth that touches the adjacent tooth.

CONVEX — curving outward.

CREST — a prominence or ridge; the height.

CUSP — an elevation on the crown of the tooth.

CUSP SLOPE — an inclination from the tip of the cusp to the contact area on any surface of the tooth.

DECIDUOUS (teeth) — teeth that exfoliate or shed.

DEGLUTITION — swallowing.

DENDRITE — the process that conducts impulses toward the cell body.

DENTITION — arrangement of the teeth in the dental arch.

DEVELOPMENTAL DEPRESSION — a concavity in a surface that formed while the tooth was developing.

DIPHYODONT — having two successive sets of teeth.

DISTAL — (the surface of the tooth) farthest from the midline.

DIVERGENT — spread.

EFFERENT — the nerves that carry motor messages away from the brain.

EMBRASURE — a curvature on the tooth that allows the food to spill away (spillway).

EMINENCE — a prominence.

ERUPTION — the moving of the tooth occlusally.

EXFOLIATE — to shed.

EXTERNAL — on the outer surface.

FACIAL — toward the face.

FISSURE — a faulty groove.

FORAMEN — an opening in a bone or hard tissue.

FORNEX — vault or arch shaped.

FOSSA — a shallow depression.

FRENUM — a fold of mucous membrane that connects two parts.

FURCATION — an area where the root trunk forks or divides.

FURROW — a groove.

GINGIVA — the mucosa that covers the alveolar bone and surrounds the teeth.

GINGIVAL CREST — the prominent edge of occlusal or incisal gingiva.

GROOVE — a long, narrow depression.

HETERODONT — different types of teeth within the same dentition (incisors, canines, molars, etc.).

HISTO-DIFFERENTIATION — development into a specialized tissue.

HISTOLOGY — the study of tissues.

HOMODONT — only one type of tooth in the dentition (i.e. all molars).

IDEAL OCCLUSION — a complete harmonious relationship of the teeth as well as other structures of the masticatory system.

INFERIOR — lower.

INSERTION — the movable end of a muscle.

INTERCUSPATION (INTERDIGITATION) — interlocking; a cusp to fossa relationship of the maxillary teeth to the mandibular teeth.

INTERNAL — within.

INTERPROXIMAL — the space between two adjoining surfaces.

INVAGINATION — to enclose within.

LABIAL — relating to the lip.

LATERAL — to the side.

LINE ANGLE — an angle formed by the joining of two surfaces.

LINGUAL — relating to the tongue.

LOBE — a major center of tooth formation.

MALOCCLUSION — any deviation from the ideal positioning of the teeth.

MAMELON — a rounded prominence on the incisal edge of newly erupted incisors which are remnants of lobe formation.

MANDIBULAR — relating to the lower jaw or mandible.

MARGINAL RIDGE — a linear elevation located around the perimeter of a surface.

MASTICATION — chewing.

MASTICATORY SYSTEM — teeth and surrounding structures: jaws, temporomandibular joint, muscles, lips, tongue, and related nerves and blood vessels.

MATRIX — a basic substance from which something forms.

MAXILLARY — relating to the upper jaw or maxilla.

MEDIAL — near the middle or medial plane.

MELANIN — a dark pigment.

MENTAL — relating to the chin.

MESIAL — toward the middle.

MODIOLUS — an area of intertwining muscles.

MORPHODIFFERENTIATION — development into specific form or structure.

MORPHOLOGY — the study of form or structure.

MUCOSA — mucous membrane.

NASAL — relating to the nose.

NEURON — a nerve cell.

OBLIQUE RIDGE — a linear elevation that transverses a surface.

OCCLUDE — to close the teeth together.

OCCLUSAL — relating to the biting surface.

OCCLUSION — the relationship of the maxillary and mandibular arch in a closed position.

ORAL CAVITY — the mouth.

ORIGIN — the fixed end of a muscle.

PASSIVE ERUPTION — the increased exposure of the tooth. As a person ages, the gingiva recedes so that the clinical crown is greater.

PERIODONTIUM — the structures that surround and support the teeth.

PERMANENT TEETH — the teeth that replace the deciduous or primary teeth.

PIT — a pinpoint depression.

PLICA — a fold of tissue.

POINT ANGLE — the area on the tooth where three surfaces meet.

POLYPHYODONT — having several sets of teeth during a lifespan.

POSTERIOR — toward the back.

PREFUNCTION ERUPTION — see active eruption.

PRIMATE SPACING — the normal spacing between primary anterior teeth.

PROLIFERATION — rapid reproduction.

PROXIMAL — nearest the point of attachment; the mesial or distal surface of the tooth.

PROXIMAL SURFACE — the surface of the tooth adjacent to the next tooth or the mesial and distal surfaces.

PULP CANAL — the portion of the pulp in the root of the tooth.

PULP CAVITY — the entire space within the tooth that contains pulp tissue.

PULP CHAMBER — the portion of the pulp in the crown of the tooth.

PULP HORN — the portion of the pulp chamber that extends toward a cusp.

QUADRANT — a fourth (of the dentition).

RAPHE — a union of soft tissue.

RESORB — to dissolve into the tissue.

RIDGE — a linear elevation.

ROOT TRUNK — that portion of the root that is not bifurcated or trifurcated.

SOCKET — a cavity in the bone; see alveolus.

SOMATIC — nerves that supply muscles.

SPILLWAY — see embrasure.

SUCCEDANEOUS — a tooth that replaces or succeeds another tooth.

SULCUS — a shallow depression.

SUPERIOR — higher or above.

SUPERNUMERARY — exceeding a fixed number.

SUTURE — a joining of two bones.

SYMMETRICAL — exact form of both sides of a dividing line.

TERMINAL MESIAL STEP — the position of a vertical plane along the distal surfaces when the deciduous second molars are in Class I position.

TERMINAL PLANE — the distal surfaces of the maxillary and mandibular deciduous second molars are on the same line or plane.

TRANSVERSE RIDGE — a linear elevation that crosses a surface (usually the occlusal surface).

TRIANGULAR RIDGE — a linear elevation that forms a triangle.

TRIFURCATION — forked or divided into three (roots).

TUBERCLE — a small, rounded projection.

TUBEROSITY — a large, rounded projection.

UNIVERSAL — common to all purposes.

VERMILION — red.

VISCERAL — nerves that supply internal organs (viscera).

Bibliography

Ash, Major. *Wheeler's Dental Anatomy, Physiology and Occlusion.* Philadelphia: Saunders, 1984.

Barrett, Richard H., and Marvin L. Hanson. *Oral Myofunctional Disorders.* 2nd ed. Saint Louis: C.V. Mosby Company, 1978.

Brand, Richard, and Donald Isselhard. *Anatomy of Orofacial Structures.* St. Louis: C.V. Mosby Co., 1982.

Carranza, Fermar. *Glickman's Clinical Periodontology.* Philadelphia: Saunders, 1984.

D.A.E. Project. *Oral Inspection I.* Teachers College Press, Columbia University, NY, 1982.

DeAngelis, Vincent, D.M.D. *Dentofacial Growth and Development; Orthodontics.* Dental Auxiliary Practice Module 2, Williams and Wilkins, 1975.

Fried, Lawrence A. *Anatomy of Head, Neck, Face and Jaws.* 2nd ed. Philadelphia: Lea and Febiger, 1980.

Fuller, James, and Gerald Denehy. *Concise Dental Anatomy and Morphology.* Chicago: Year Book Medical Publishers, 1977.

Gray, Henry. *Anatomy of the Human Body.* Edited by Charles Mayo Goss. 29th ed. Philadelphia: Lea and Febiger, 1973.

Hosl, E. et al. *Orthodontics and Periodontics.* Chicago: Quintessence Publishing Co., 1985.

Massler, M., and J. Schour. *Atlas of the Mouth.* Chicago: American Dental Association, 1975.

Melfi, Rudy. *Permar's Oral Embryology and Microscopic Anatomy.* Philadelphia: Lea and Febiger, 1982.

Moss-Salentijn, L., and M. Hendricks-Klyvert. *Dental and Oral Tissues, An Introduction.* Philadelphia: Lea and Febiger, 1985.

Orban's Oral Histology and Embryology. Edited by S.N. Bhaskar. 8th ed. Saint Louis: C.V. Mosby Company, 1976.

Oregon State System. *Dental Anatomy, A Self-instructional Program.* Norwalk, CT: Appleton-Century Crofts, 1982.

Phillips, R. *Elements of Dental Material for Dental Hygienists and Dental Assistants.* Philadelphia: Saunders, 1984.

Ramfjord, S., and M. Ash. *Occlusion.* Philadelphia: Saunders, 1983.

Reed, G., and V. Sheppard. *Basic Structures of the Head and Neck*. Philadelphia: Saunders, 1976.

Riviere, Holliston L. *Anatomy and Embryology of the Head and Neck*. Reston, VA: Reston Publishing Company, 1983.

Sassouni, V., and E. Forrest. *Orthodontics in Dental Practice*. St. Louis: C.V. Mosby, 1971.

Shapiro, H. *Maxillofacial Anatomy*. Philadelphia: Lippincott, 1954.

Wheeler, R. *An Atlas of Tooth Form*. Philadelphia: W.B. Saunders, 1984.

Wheeler, R. *Textbook of Dental Anatomy and Physiology*. Philadelphia: W.B. Saunders, 1965.

Wilkins, Esther M. *Clinical Practice of the Dental Hygienist*. Philadelphia: Lea and Febiger, 1983.

Woelfel, Julian B. *Dental Anatomy: Its Correlation with Dental Health Service*. 3rd ed. Philadelphia: Lea and Febiger, 1984.

Woodall, Irene et al. *Comprehensive Dental Hygiene Care*. St. Louis: C.V. Mosby, 1985.

INDEX